Doctors on the Edge

DOCTORS ON THE EDGE

will your doctor break the rules for you?

FREDRICK R. ABRAMS, M.D.

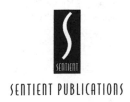

SENTIENT PUBLICATIONS

Cover design by Kim Johansen
Book design by Timm Bryson

All names, identifying characteristics, and other details
have been altered to protect patient privacy.

Library of Congress Cataloging-in-Publication Data

Abrams, Fredrick R.
  Doctors on the edge : will your doctor break the rules for you? / Fredrick R. Abrams.
     p. ; cm.
  Includes bibliographical references.
  ISBN-13: 978-1-59181-045-2
  ISBN-10: 1-59181-045-0
  1. Medical ethics. 2. Physicians--Professional ethics. I. Title.
  [DNLM: 1. Ethics, Medical. W 50 A161d 2006]
  R725.5.A27 2006
  174.2--dc22

                          2006017951

Printed in the United States of America

10 9 8 7 6 5 4 3 2 1

SENTIENT PUBLICATIONS, LLC
1113 Spruce Street
Boulder, CO 80302
www.sentientpublications.com

*To the person whose opinion of me
and my work I value above all others,
my best friend and first reader, my wife*

Alice M. Abrams

TABLE *of* CONTENTS

A PHYSICIAN'S AFFIRMATION

In order to be worthy of self-respect, I pledge to give the respect due to others who place their trust in me as a professional in the healing arts. Therefore:

I will practice my art and my science to benefit my patients.

I will disclose to my patients that which I know of their disease, and any hazards of the remedies I might suggest, so that I may guide them to choose the course that suits them best.

I will offer care and comfort when they are ill, and when death becomes inevitable, I will ease their way as best I can in keeping with their expressed plan.

I will recognize their right to self-determination, and if a conflict should arise with my own ethical constraints, I will make them aware without judging wherein we differ so that they may consider seeking help elsewhere for their complaints.

I will intercede in their behalf within the scope of my authority if I perceive they are being treated without regard for their humanity.

I will hold in confidence that which is seen or heard in my role as physician.

I will ever be a student, sharpening my skills and knowledge to make me a better clinician

If I act in this way, I may aspire to join the men and women who through the ages have approached the loftiest ideals of the healing mission, for I will have earned the faith and trust that is the strongest tie in the bond between patient and physician.

—Fredrick Ralph Abrams, M.D.

INTRODUCTION

Often, "doctor stories" are anecdotes of spectacular cures, split-second interventions dramatized on video, or documentaries of life-and-limb-saving technology. Less is heard about the human dilemmas, decisions, and quiet actions that also change lives (or sometimes forestall unwanted change)—of stories recounting the daily moral challenges for a profession where both body and soul are laid bare.

The narratives here are in a medical setting, but the problems are universal: grindingly painful illnesses, marital infidelity, aging parents, end-of-life decisions, gender confusion, infertility with its irrational feelings of inadequacy, and socially devastating secrets—the exigencies of being human. The often-told melodramatic "hero stories" are frequently preselected to leave no doubt that what was done was the "right thing to do." The stories I will relate do not have that air of certainty about them. A dilemma often has more than one ethically defensible response and always leaves you wondering.

Medical education is so crowded with "must know" facts, figures, and techniques that only occasionally does the training venture into human values. Too little time is allotted for rumination on which values are "right." Medical practice is concerned with what works, which treatment is most likely to result in the greatest medical benefit. Philosophers label that ethical approach to problems "utilitarianism," focused on action and the outcome it spawns. Timeliness of interventions is often critical. There are four minutes to restore oxygen to the brain from the time a heart stops before permanent damage results. Medical staff must respond quickly. They must often take action based on incomplete information. If the emergency room (ER) doctor were confronted with an unknown patient with cardiac arrest, resuscitation would be attempted on the principle "when in doubt, err on the side of life." Had the doctor known that the cardiac arrest resulted from widespread and incurable cancer, she would have made no futile attempts at resuscitation. But because important facts are lacking and consequences are not always predictable, moral decisions must be made on the spot, according to experience and the bias of an individual's values.

Most physicians hold values that have been incorporated into their behavior before they arrive at medical school. Regard for the truth, inclination to help the less fortunate, putting self-interest aside, prioritizing sanctity or quality of life—these are difficult values to teach to an adult who has not already integrated them into his or her character. Experience in and after medical school may serve to affirm or modify the morality they have brought to their chosen profession. There is no code to which laypersons can refer to predict how any individual doctor will respond to requests for abortion or pleas for euthanasia or assisted suicide, or how she will react to a patient's alternative sexual lifestyle.

For over twenty years, I have been concerned with the way medicine, law, and morality become entwined, and how they then, uninvited and unexpected, intrude on everyday private lives. The questions of right and wrong are always with us and need constant weighing and balancing. These stories may help people to analyze situations in which, no matter which choice is made, some good will be left undone or some evil will be perpetuated. That is why ethics has been called "the logic of tragedy."

No one will meet all of these situations in their lifetime, but everyone can take away something of value from contemplating moral dilemmas. The mental exercise will stand them in good stead should they encounter quandaries of their own. I also encourage readers, in advance of a crisis, to consider how they might deal with these problems and to engage their doctors in serious conversation about personal values. There are some specific ethical underpinnings of medical practice—the codes and guidelines, theories and principles that aid but do not spell out decisions for doctors and patients. They are corrals within which ethical decisions may be found rather than paths leading directly to the right answer. Moral compatibility with doctors is essential in order for patients to receive the kind of treatment they desire. Everyone experiences the periods of human transition; birth and genetics (with tragedies of abnormal births and developmental disability), sexuality (within and outside of marriage), reproductive successes and failures, illnesses and aging, attitude and gratitude between parents and children, and death and dying—and all are fraught with medical-moral decisions.

Doctors, if they wish, may become mere technicians, offering their skills and knowledge as a commodity—simply selling whatever the patient wishes to buy. Very little ethical judgment need be employed. For some, it is easier that way. The stories I will relate are not about doctors who simply provided their technical skills. They are about doctors who went beyond that role in an effort to bring about what they believed to be the best outcome for their patients. But in so doing, they sometimes lied, betrayed confidences, or broke or stretched the law.

You will find some of them difficult to condemn and some difficult to condone. A few of them anticipated changes in the law that simply came about too slowly. Philosophers who contemplate certain injustices in the world often advise against precipitous action. Especially, they urge adhering to the law and social convention. They recommend instead "working within the system" to make changes where they seem to be needed. They fear unacceptable social unrest should everyone ignore the rules of society. But periodically one encounters a situation that calls for anticipation of changes in law and policy that are in the wind but grind too slowly through the legal mill. Extant laws are broken, it's true, but in the patient's interest and in anticipation of a wiser resolution in the future.

If you feel these actions were justified, you must ask yourself why. What is different about the lapses from conventional ethical behavior in these stories? How are they distinguished from other ethical deviations, from deceptions that you would quickly and firmly condemn?

Do you agree that doctors and patients may make choices that violate conventional ethics and can be the best of anguishing alternatives? Or do you believe the actions these doctors took were simply wrong? Where are the limits to bending laws, rules, or the truth?

In reviewing these events, the reader may often discern elements of paternalism, but in no case were measures undertaken solely for the doctor's benefit. When these doctors measured the consequences for patients or others, no patient was deceived or exploited, nor was any person treated as an object only. The stories are true, but the names, locations, and sometimes the age or gender—in fact, all identifying factors—are not true. I speak in the voice of the doctors and patients to whom these stories belong. They are not all my stories, although I tell almost all of them in first person as they or their doctor told them to me, using literary license to speculate on thoughts and emotions that were not always actually voiced. I have adopted this device because I am familiar with many of these situations. I have met similar dilemmas. I accept my share of the guilt that sometimes comes with violations of conventional ethics because I agree with most of the actions taken. I believe all were taken with the intention of benefiting the patients involved.

THE TRUTH
ABOUT ANDREA

Although six years have gone by, the experience was so extraordinary that I recall every detail of Andrea's first appointment. I remember blocking extra time for her consultation, anticipating the complexity of that introductory visit. Despite cautioning myself to be nonchalant and objective, as Andrea stepped into my consulting room, the savoir faire I had intended to project and had rehearsed in my mind dissolved in an instant. I was astonished! No resolve could stem the flush in my cheeks that betrayed my amazement. I stood and reached across my desk to shake the hand of the groomed, poised, and attractive young woman who entered. Her surgeon, one of very few who offers the intricate and arduous surgery of gender change, had called me about the referral a week before. Despite more than two decades of gynecological practice, this was my first encounter, personally (insofar as I knew) or professionally, with a patient born a male who was now a female.

After the surgeon's call, as I reviewed the hormone treatment necessary to maintain a transsexual's feminine contour, the visceral nature of my bias crept into my consciousness. I had resolved, despite all my reservations, that when Andrea kept her appointment I was going to comport myself with the objectivity of the dispassionate scientist and the sincere empathy of the consummate physician.

Upon first seeing Andrea, I thought fleetingly that someone had rearranged my schedule. There was nothing of the "drag queen" about her, no caricature of femininity. She was—simply a woman.

Her appearance was vastly different from the stereotypical image I had conjured in my imagination. No shadow of a badly disguised beard. No stentorian voice. How insidiously prejudice had penetrated my professional veneer! Would my medical training have permitted me to pick her out from other gynecology patients in the waiting room, had I not been forewarned? I was chagrined to admit that it would not. I was ashamed and fearful that my ineptly camouflaged bias had been transparent to Andrea, a person who had suffered yet endured prejudice and who most needed my help and acceptance.

Over the ensuing six years that we spent as doctor and patient, my negative bias dissipated as I saw that her behavior, aspirations, and daily tribulations were no different from those of my other patients. As she began to trust me, she recalled the torment of her feelings of alienation when she was a young boy and the ambivalence of adolescence. When she was in her twenties, she became certain she had been assigned the wrong body, and she seized the courage to begin medical consultations.

No doctor will do sex reassignment without extensive evaluation. Surgery is permanent. No one wants to be a party to operating on a transvestite who simply wishes to dress in women's clothes; for such a person, surgery would be a tragedy, confusing him with a committed transsexual for whom surgery is the ultimate empowerment.

For almost two years as part of her doctor's conditions, Andrea practiced being a female by changing jobs, cross-dressing, and essentially being a woman. During this time, despite politically correct protestations that men and women are treated alike in the workplace and socially, Andrea experienced the actual differences and found that she liked them. Daily habits, patterns of speech, manners, and behavior that defined her as a woman became second nature—or perhaps first nature—to her.

Preoperative hormone therapy helped her become a new self as her breasts began to develop and a contour pleasing to her materialized as fat redistributed around the hips. Her skin became smoother, and arduous inch-by-inch electrolysis completed the task, eliminating facial hair. She found these changes to be rewarding and enjoyed the fanciful thought of herself as a butterfly emerging from a chrysalis. The health insurance she had at work gave partial coverage for the very expensive surgical, medical, and psychological consultations and procedures. She told me about the more mundane barriers she had struggled through that I hadn't even thought about. Changing a single letter in her name, which had been Andrew, transformed it from masculine to feminine, but it needed an official imprimatur, as did her birth certificate and her driver's license—the daily bureaucracy that all of us endure but surmount with much less red tape, and without the raised eyebrows and scornful looks that she confronted. Finally, she had made the surgical rectification. She was happy.

On a later visit, Andrea disclosed that she had never divulged to her husband the specifics of her surgery or of her former life; she also cautioned me not to expose her medical history inadvertently should her husband ever accompany her to the office. I did not comment after she offered this information, but I suspect the quizzical expression that involuntarily appeared on my face prompted her to explain to me the painful prelude to her decision to withhold the whole truth from her husband.

Earlier, there had been another man with whom her relationship had become serious. After nearly a year of progressive intimacy, both emotional and physical, she tormented herself pondering the heartbreak of rejection that might ensue if she revealed her past. The decision to disclose it was precipitated by his proposal of marriage; she felt she could no longer procrastinate. She entrusted her extraordinary history to him. After short-lived disbelief, he had fled in a state of massive confusion, wrestling with the inference of homosexuality that, to him, his attraction to her had implied. Andrea, bruised by the emotional devastation honesty had wrought, decided to reveal to the man who would ultimately become her husband only that she was unable to have children. They had agreed that they would pursue adoption when their relationship felt secure enough for them to raise a child. Now, happily married for three years, they want to adopt children and live the family life to which many men and women aspire.

Most of my patients consider adoption only after they have

undergone exhaustive diagnostic procedures and repeated failures of treatment, reluctantly surrendering to the reality that they can neither conceive nor bear a child. Andrea had run a different gauntlet. She had been born a male and lived "in quiet desperation" as a boy and a man for twenty-two years. After a decade of humiliating experiences and fervent self-examination, with professional counseling she had undergone the gender-changing surgery. At last, she assumed the body she perceived she had been denied at birth, and she shed the male trappings with which she felt she had mistakenly been burdened.

Andrea brought with her an "Application for Adoption" and begged me to fill it out without revealing the extraordinary—and to some people, abominable—details of her operation. The questionnaire (all spaces must be filled in) demanded to know whether she had had any previous surgery, and if so, to describe it. Certainly, it's a legitimate question to ask when the health of adoptive parents may diminish their ability to care for a child. Yet there must be a way to answer the question that would not disqualify her in too many biased minds from parenting by adoption.

There is a myth about an unprovoked assault on an inoffensive cherry tree by a Founding Father that credulous American children are raised upon, and I was among them. "I cannot tell a lie." But right at that moment, Andrea was asking me, her doctor, to falsify a medical record—and I wanted to find a way. My thoughts slithered into the dark and shadowy corners of my mind where creative mendacity lurks.

The Hippocratic tradition is that doctors take care of their patients almost as a parent cares for a child. Confidentiality is specified in the Oath that bears this ancient physician's name: "What I may see or hear in the course of treatment...which on no account one must spread abroad, I will keep to myself, holding such things to be shameful to be spoken about." Nevertheless, doctors are expected to fill out honestly numerous privacy-invading forms that characterize modern medical practice. Dilemmas have a special characteristic—no matter which decision is made, some evil will be done or some good will be lost, simultaneously and unavoidably. In this case, either to lie or to disclose the facts would have those characteristics.

What's a lie?[1] Most dictionaries define it as a *false* statement made with the deliberate intention to deceive. The secondary definitions refer to *anything* that includes an intent to deceive; it need not be false per se. Why should we agonize over lying? Communication between individuals is what creates the "social" part of a society. If lies and truths were randomly mingled, there could be no social order, no cooperation. It's clear, however, that a smile or a wink can be just as perfidious as a spoken lie. We concede there are times when truth can cause at least as much damage as a lie, so we provide for prevarication. Perhaps all lies are wrong, but some can be forgiven. We call them "white lies." However, we insist on rules that say lies must be justified, while the truth stands on its own. Just as the Eskimos have many more words for snow than we do, because subtle differences have great significance for their survival, so well over one hundred synonyms and variations may be found for *lie*.[2] Our society needs abundant words for lies if we're going to survive.

For many doctors, there's a premise more fundamental than truth. From ancient medical writings called the *Hippocratic Corpus* (not the Oath), comes the admonition, "First, do no harm." If the first objective with patients—the basic value—is to do them no harm, truth may be shaded or shunted in the interest of avoiding harm. Dipping into the tangled web of deception, doctors with benevolent intentions bring forth panoplies of lies. How can such deviation from conventional ethics be constrained to avoid a total breakdown of communication? There are mandatory elements to justify deception. Lying can never be included in the moral structure of medicine unless it is done on behalf of the patient. The harms must be balanced and proportionate. The doctor's and the patient's concept of harm must be in accord. Serious injury or exploitation of others must be avoided.

Would Andrea make a good mother? Indeed, I asked myself, what makes a mother good? What is the best interest of the child to be adopted? There was very little precedent to guide me. No license is needed to procreate. Much of it is accidental. How can we measure the ingredients for a good adoption? We've all seen "good" kids come from "bad" homes and "bad" kids come from "good" homes.

Concerning Andrea's relationship with the rest of the world, I was already a conspirator. Did I have to answer the agency's question truthfully? The purpose of the question was to determine if Andrea's health permits her be physically and emotionally capable of raising a child. A detailed answer could introduce a bias that ought have no place in the decision.

And most critical of all, in this specific instance, what was significantly true about Andrea, her husband, and parenting? I felt I knew Andrea and her husband as well as any professional with frequent but limited contact can know another. Although doctor visits are relatively short, they can be extremely intense. The social niceties that limit intimacy in other venues are often dispensed with in the doctor's office. I had been privy to discussions about their marriage, lifestyles, values, and aspirations. I had listened to the hardships she had undergone so she might achieve what she considered the epitome of womanhood; namely, home and family. I knew, from Andrea, about the conditions they had set with each other for adoption, but I had not spoken to her husband about them. This visit, he accompanied her to the office. I invited him in to talk about his feelings about adoption. The three of us exchanged ideas for almost an hour. I was convinced they were aware of the complexity of child rearing and had thought long and hard about it. I confess to a degree of arrogance as I decided what to write, but it was accompanied by a heartfelt hope that it was the right thing. I looked at the form and filled it out while they waited. When it came to the question about surgery, the facts were there, but the truth was obscured behind a screen of medical jargon. I made no false statement.

PAST SURGERY [LIST OPERATIONS]
(1) Resection for a benign congenital condition resulting in extirpation of the gonads with resulting infertility.

(They need not be told the benign congenital condition was possession of male sexual organs.)

CURRENT MEDICATIONS [INDICATION]
(1) Hormone replacement therapy

(They need not be told it was replacement of male testosterone by female estrogen.)

How would the agency's committee translate these statements?

- Resection—surgical removal
- Benign—not a cancer
- Congenital condition—anything a person is born with
- Extirpate—another word for complete surgical removal
- Gonads—reproductive organs (ovaries in a female, testes in a male)

Anyone interviewing Andrea would see an attractive female. From her written medical history, the inference would be that she was born with abnormal female organs necessitating removal of her uterus and ovaries, rendering her infertile and necessitating estrogen replacement. And, to tell the truth(!), that's all they needed to know.

ASK ME NO QUESTIONS

If there were a reality television program called "Spot the Adulteress," no one would pick Laura out of the lineup to brand with the scarlet letter. She did not look the part. When Laura was in the company of other adults, she was invisible. Only when she was addressed directly would she answer, and then in a barely audible voice. Parent-teacher nights were agony, which she endured only because the conversation related to her cherished pupils. Some parents of new kindergartners invariably expressed misgivings to the principal, fearful because their child's first teacher appeared to be so ineffective. But those who pursued their concerns by auditing their child's classes quickly dismissed their reservations as they watched Laura minister to her little students. When she was shepherding the children, some singular alchemy transmuted her timidity into a golden gentleness. Her knack of bolstering the fragile egos of her malleable charges was first among the talents that enabled her to be the exemplary teacher that she was. The children adored her. Once she was home, she spent every spare minute with the two boys of her own. Nurturing the children exhausted her energy, leaving little at the end of the day for her husband, Stuart.

Despite her reticence, Laura is attractive with fine features, albeit scrupulously devoid of makeup. A severe hairstyle and round, steel-rimmed glasses completes the disguise. In the romantic movie cliché, such a character suddenly undergoes a transformation: a new hairstyle, makeup, an enticing gown, and lo! The duckling vanishes and the swan appears. Except Laura never did the makeover.

She as the patient and I as her obstetrician found ourselves mired in a dilemma. We had little time for reflection as we struggled to deal with a devastating truth. We made instant choices around which both our futures pivoted. Brushing aside conventional ethics, I chose to join Laura in a lie and, further, to falsify official records.

On my "night of the lies," the phone jangled me into consciousness, and I snatched it from its cradle. The answering service patched the message through, noting it was an emergency. Laura was calling. It was out of character for her to phone so late. She could barely squeeze the words out.

"I'm—in the car. Stuart's driving me—to the emergency room."

"What's wrong?"

"Pain—I have—a horrible pain—in my side; I dreamed—I was a little girl —running and running. I heard—mother's voice—shrieking all around me, 'I warned you, I warned you.' I tripped—the scissors stuck into me. It felt like—my insides—were burning. I thought, *This is a dream. Wake up!* But the pain didn't go away. Something is ripping my insides."

Half awake and confused, I asked, "What about a scissors?"

"No, that's the dream—but the pain—it's still there."

Responding to the urgency in her voice, without pursuing more information I said, "Okay, I'll meet you."

I dressed hurriedly, trying to recall conversations I had had with Laura. When her second pregnancy was diagnosed, she had become agitated. She volunteered that being pregnant was not a joyful surprise, not a blessed event for her upcoming thirty-fifth birthday. She was concerned about how Stuart would react.

"Stuart and I talked about another baby back when Chrissie was two," she remembered. "We were watching TV and there were two children playing, so I asked Stuart if he thought we might have another baby to keep Chrissie company. He told me we couldn't afford it. Even raising one is tough, especially now with colleges getting so expensive. Y' know Stuart's always been in charge of the money. He's a CPA," she reminded me. "So what he says about money is mostly the way it goes. He's usually right, so it's okay with me."

Laura reflected that she hadn't thought much about having

another child before TV cued the question, although I suspect it had been lurking not far below the surface. Stuart had considered the idea but had vetoed it on economic grounds. He always constructed his arguments carefully, as fit the personality of a CPA who had to deal meticulously with rigid rules and mathematical certainties. Indeed, this mind-set was the essence of his character. Boundaries were to be honored, and rules were to be followed. "For Stuart," Laura complained, "it's not really the risk of bending rules; you just don't do it; it's inexcusable."

Their first child had been carefully planned to arrive after five years of marriage, when Stuart had calculated they could afford a baby. Laura and Stuart alike treasured Christopher. Laura had settled well into the single-child routine they had chosen. The unplanned second pregnancy after a five-year hiatus threw them off balance at first. After the initial surprise, Laura admitted to a certain satisfaction with the pregnancy. Although Stuart was not famous for flexibility, he did some recalculating and agreed that they need make only minor adjustments in their lifestyle. Abortion never entered the equation. Before long, Stuart waxed enthusiastic and became devoted to the new baby. He quickly joined the trend and became a hands-on father, changing Noah's diapers and backpacking him on the family expeditions (which were always planned to avoid tax season). He thought of his family as a successful balance sheet, with each integer contributing to the sum, immutably in its proper place, taken for granted. Following the birth, Laura had returned to her teaching job as soon as she felt strong enough. It was essential to her definition of herself, and they truly needed the income.

During that last pregnancy, Stuart wanted to be certain there would be no more miscalculations in their life plan as he had structured it, so we three had a discussion about permanent birth control. I was pleased that they chose to sit side by side on a small sofa in my office, passing up two separate chairs across from me. Laura asked about "Band-Aid" sterilization for herself. Stuart unconsciously placed his arm around her protectively.

I recommended instead that they consider surgery for Stuart, a vasectomy. It could be done under local anesthesia, with small, super-ficial incisions and a direct view of the ducts to be severed. Infection or injury to other organs is rare. The operation on Laura, named after the "Band-Aid" dressing that could completely cover the small inci-sion, nevertheless risked damaging the bowel or bladder, or lacerat-ing a major blood vessel. Anesthesia needs to be deeper, and the chance of infection is greater.

They agreed that neither wished to parent another child, regard-less of what the future held. When Stuart heard about the differences in the risks for the surgical options, to his credit he had immediately agreed to a vasectomy. When he volunteered for the operation, Laura reached up to squeeze the almost paternal hand that lay across her shoulder, and a smile flashed across Stuart's face in response. Driving to the hospital, I remembered that Stuart had had his "tubes tied" even before the delivery of Noah.

Stuart was pacing nervously in the waiting room. Anxiously, he grasped my arm, propelling me urgently toward the curtained door. "Laura's in the exam room," he explained unnecessarily. Hurrying through the doorway, I almost collided with a lab tech leaving with a blood sample for a blood count and cross matching, should a trans-fusion be necessary. I heard the beep-beep of the pulse monitor, which was ominously fast, even before I saw Laura lying on the exam-ination table. She was clutching the sheets, knuckles white, eyes half shut. Intravenous fluid was dripping into her arm from a clear plastic bag. Her abdomen was rigid to the touch, and the pain was greatest on the left side, ruling out appendicitis. Being a gynecologist, I asked about menstrual periods. She was uncertain. Since Stuart's vasecto-my, she hadn't felt the need to keep close track of her cycles, she said, avoiding my eyes.

After years of practice, I had learned to become suspicious with a patient's uncertainty about menstrual history. Before abortions were legal, a teenager once came to my office bleeding profusely. As I examined her, I saw protruding from her uterus a rubber tube that had been used to interrupt an early pregnancy. I removed it and showed it to her. She asked, "What is that, and how did it get there?"

eyes wide open in feigned astonishment. Such events prepare you to regard questions and answers with skeptical optimism.

Patients become extremely agitated if their fidelity is challenged. Apologizing for asking, I pressed ahead. The information I needed was too important for me to be squeamish about hurt feelings. "Stuart had a vasectomy, but could you be pregnant anyway?" I inquired as gently as I could.

"Yes!" erupted so suddenly I was startled.

Her face reddened, and the blush spread to her neck as she related her story. I pieced the scene together from sentence fragments blurted spasmodically through clenched teeth and tears. An attentive and handsome young assistant principal had on several occasions assured her that passing her thirty-fifth birthday hadn't marked the end of her feminine attractiveness. The Stuart she loved had always been a responsible husband, but never a responsive one. As in any marriage, compromises were made, but the longings couldn't be erased. For the first time in a decade, someone was paying her exclusive and flattering attention. Feelings were reawakened that had long subsided in the routine of marriage, work, and child rearing. One day, the babysitter had been asked to stay later because of Laura's mandatory late-night teacher's program. The program coincided with her husband's extended absence during tax season. Stuart virtually lived at the office, January to April fifteenth.

Rashly, she accepted the invitation of the attractive younger man for a drink at his home after the program. Seduced by his flattering attention and assurances of her desirability, and with the aid of two Manhattans, she had succumbed to his gentle but persistent advances, more in gratitude than in passion. Contraception had not been Laura's concern since Stuart's vasectomy. And the school principal's crowd had always left that issue to the more sophisticated young women in his circle.

Overwhelmed with guilt and remorse, she immediately made it clear to her paramour that this unconscionable blunder would never happen again. And it didn't.

In a rush of words, she poured out the neediness she had been feeling in her marriage. She sobbed of her love for Stuart but also of her disappointment. It simply wasn't part of Stuart's nature to recognize and respond to her craving for unsolicited small attentions and appreciation. She pleaded for understanding, seeking from me absolution that was not mine to give. Over and over again, she urged me to believe that this single instance has been the only episode of infidelity in ten years of marriage. How deeply she wished it had never happened!

The diagnosis of pregnancy was confirmed with a two-minute urine test. The two minutes seemed like hours as I listened to the increasingly rapid beeping of the monitor. I saw the bright pulse line rising as the blood pressure fell, fearful that the lines would cross, signaling imminent catastrophe. The pain and bleeding strongly indicated that the pregnancy was in the fallopian tube, not the womb. This pregnancy would be unable to progress.

An egg fertilized in the ovary must traverse the delicate, pencil-sized fallopian tube on its journey to the womb, where it has room to grow. If it straggles on its voyage and implants instead in the wall of the tube, it will grow there until it bursts its narrow confines, rending the fragile tissues and the surrounding blood vessels. This is a life-threatening accident. Surgery is necessary to prevent a fatal hemorrhage.

The pregnancy test confirmed Laura's worst fear. Her only thought was how to avoid revealing to Stuart that she was pregnant. Certain that the truth would result in divorce and permanent separation from her children, she could not begin to consider the alarming medical condition she faced. The threat that her single episode of infidelity would be revealed concerned her more than the bleeding in her abdomen. I explained that the pregnancy would never come to term. It was already miscarrying, but it was implanted in a dangerous place, rupturing tissue and blood vessels. Surgery without delay was critical.

She was not listening to me. "I know him," she forced through clenched teeth. "He'd never forgive me." Again, I tried to explain, but she wouldn't listen. "Please, please, don't tell him. He'll take the children."

She might have been right. I thought about previous talks with her and Stuart. Mistakes are not allowable in his world. In his eyes, she would be a mother unfit to raise his children. His unyielding values about rules and order might indeed have led to what she feared, even more than her death. My precipitous judgment was that Stuart would not be able to withstand a simultaneous assault on his ego and on his value system. Was that an outcome that could truly be anticipated, or was I being swept into the wild imaginings of a guilt-ridden, overwhelmed mother?

There was no time for a lengthy discussion—for the type of cautious and protracted counseling that might have enabled us to slip gently into the truth, to test the water without taking the plunge. If we had had the luxury of time, perhaps Stuart might have been eased into the truth. I could not dwell long on Laura's fears of the future, however, because it is always the critical present that must be confronted.

It's easier to tell the truth. That still, small voice says, "People must be responsible for their actions. You don't know what Stuart will do. You can only guess. If the outcome for their marriage is bad, that's their problem. You shouldn't violate the universal obligation to tell the truth. It is sheer arrogance to believe you can predict the future and solve everyone's problems better than they can themselves, if they know the truth."

"Do no harm," counters the time-honored aphorism. Was the consequence she feared predictable enough to warrant my conspiracy with Laura? That was what had to be quickly decided. Moreover, I would have to falsify hospital records, risking my medical license and my livelihood as well. That factor was undeniably crucial to my decision. How could I rush Laura to surgery without an explanation to Stuart? Was there any way out of her nightmare? I knew I could not suborn all the witnesses (the emergency room personnel, operating room nurses, and the anesthesiologist) to a deception. A second chance for Laura? I had to believe she was telling the truth. I had to believe that the situation was just as she presented it. I had to believe that this had been a single lapse. Time was rushing by. I had to believe!

Her increasingly rapid pulse indicated blood was leaking out of the system that carries life-sustaining oxygen to the brain. The heart was laboring to compensate by pushing the diminished blood volume faster. Only after explaining my plan to Laura did she consent to surgery. I confess that if she hadn't agreed, I would have forced the surgery upon her. Justifying the use of force to operate without consent would have been easier than risking the consequence of honoring her refusal. Alone now in the examining room with her, I took the laboratory report of the pregnancy test out of the chart, folded it carefully, and put it in my pocket. We had become conspirators.

Our course was resolved, and swiftly we brought Laura to the operating room. The entire interval since my arrival at the emergency room had been compressed into fifteen anxious minutes. En route, I hastily told Stuart a half truth, "There appears to be internal bleeding, and immediate surgery must be done to prevent a fatal hemorrhage." I did not divulge the probable cause, excusing myself with the proposition that I really didn't know with certainty, yet. The anesthesiologist was waiting. It had been over eight hours since Laura had eaten, so she could be put to sleep safely with general anesthesia.

The nurses washed her abdomen with antiseptics. Then, after I scrubbed, they handed me sterile towels to surround the site around where the incisions would be, leaving only a small window that allowed access to her abdomen. A long, sterile sheet with a carefully cut hole fit neatly over my towels, isolating the site for surgery. As much as shielding Laura from infection, the sheet shielded her from me. Surgical drapes were created to assure a germ-free field, to avoid introducing infection into a wound. They serve that purpose, it is true. There is another essential effect; they remove the personality from the operating room. I didn't need to reflect on the hubris of cutting into the body of a living woman. Drapes allowed me, for the moment, to deal only with anatomy—with tissues and organs. As I was operating, I was not thinking about Laura, her two children, her husband, or her predicament. For that brief time only, during surgery, it was better that she be only a technical problem, not a vulnerable human being.

Two scissors-like clamps were ready. Instead of cutting edges, these clamps have very narrow, sharp, pincer-like ends that look like the mandibles of a gigantic ant. Grasping the skin adjacent to the navel with a shiny clamp on each side, I stretched it sideways, exposing an area for a half-inch incision within the depression. When the cut healed, it would be invisible inside the folds of skin. Next, a hollow needle was placed into the abdomen through the incision, and harmless carbon dioxide gas was allowed to flow through it. The gas expands the normally airtight abdomen so that when we pierce the skin to place our viewing scope inside, the bowel will not be pressed against the front of the belly. There would be a space allowing the abdominal contents to be examined once we inserted the periscope-like apparatus. The abdomen swelled, mocking the pregnancy that was not meant to be.

Then a long metal tube about a half inch wide was pushed through the incision. Some blood bubbled up, but the fiber optic scope with light and a lens blocked the flow as it was passed inside. This scope has an eyepiece that I look through. In this case, only I could see what the scope revealed. It was not one of those special instruments attached to a projection camera that would show everyone in the operating room images on a screen. With a thin suction tube inserted through a smaller second incision, several cups of partially clotted blood were vacuumed away, allowing me to examine the tubes and ovaries. The delicate wall of the tube was distorted by an ugly purple mass with ragged edges from which blood was steadily oozing. I saw that I would be able to arrest the blood flow without making a large, exploratory incision.

I confirmed the diagnosis of ruptured tubal pregnancy, but only to myself. To the operating room staff, I lied, "There's a bleeder in a ruptured ovary." I evacuated the disrupted pregnancy using the small suction tube. The quarter teaspoon of formless, fragmented tissue that was an incipient pregnancy joined imperceptibly the cups of clotted blood already in the reservoir of the suction apparatus, to be discarded. No tissue remained to be sent to the laboratory that would reveal the true diagnosis for the record. An electric current from another instrument, inserted through the small second incision, cauterized the edges of the wound, sealing the torn vessels. The bleeding stopped. She was out of danger. I asked the circulating nurse to phone the waiting room and assure Stuart that his wife was okay and tell him that I would be down soon to speak with him.

This operation removes an extremely early fetus from the mother, recognizable only under the microscope as a disrupted and formless clump of cells. Sometimes, a tubal pregnancy is detected before it ruptures. Although the surgery interrupts a pregnancy, even people who abhor abortion find terminating such pregnancies justified. Life does not always package events into neat parcels that are entirely good or exclusively bad. At this stage, it might be considered a miscarriage, not termination of a pregnancy that had potential to mature. At any stage, it can be life-threatening.

What I proposed to Laura as a way out of her predicament meant I had to lie, falsify the record, and join with Laura to deceive Stuart. After I saw Laura safely to the recovery room, I headed to the waiting room, still in scrubs, to tell Stuart part of the truth—that Laura had begun an internal hemorrhage, and we had controlled it before it became a threat to her life.

An obstetrician/gynecologist, like it or not, sees many a sunrise. Strips of sunlight were beginning to filter through the blinds as I spoke with Stuart. We were both exhausted and relieved. People who experience severe stress together bond. Feelings surface; we perceive the vulnerability all of us share. Surely, a cliché becomes a cliché because it is universally accepted, so I sermonized. I exploited the moment to reflect aloud that we never know what's in store for us, day by day. Further, this crisis underscored how important it was that we take every opportunity to demonstrate to those we love how precious they are to us, never to be taken for granted.

Stuart murmured his affirmation of that idea. He ruminated, "I'm sitting here thinking—I've been so busy trying to make money for Laura and the kids that I've ignored them. Valentines Day! I feel awful—she had a rose on my plate at dinner, and I asked what it was for. She said, 'Nothing special.' The next day—only when the receptionist asked me how many valentines did I get..." His voice trailed off, then he continued to speak disjointedly, voicing segments of his thoughts aloud, "and I didn't have the sense to say anything to her, to Laura I mean, or bring flowers then, home, that night, I mean. Y'know," he reflected, "it's been years since I brought flowers—or anything—except maybe on birthdays. Foolish! Our kids are terrific," he looked up at me, "and that's because she's such a great—mom. And I'm like, everyone has a right to expect that! What would happen—if—then my work wouldn't mean..." his voice trailed off.

Before I left the waiting room, I talked a little more about how we all value positive reinforcement, how I as a doctor would become jaded if all I received was a fee, and never any thanks from my patients. "I'm sure you value recognition from your clients, right?" I queried. I left after I suggested that expressing his appreciation to Laura would be the best outcome from this misadventure.

That evening on rounds, I reassured Laura that the surgery had gone as we had hoped, that her secret was safe. Laura had a troubled smile on her face as she said wryly, "Y'know, I really didn't need this—to reinforce the lesson plan, I mean. I'd already decided, I don't want everybody's approval all the time. Nobody should. I've got to teach that to the children. That, and that good people make mistakes. They've got to know that." She looked up. "Not that I'd talk about this," she said hastily. "My—episode—stupid episode with the principal was enough to show me how far off track—vanity—and such—dependence—could push me."

I signed the chart out as hemorrhagic ovarian cyst, with no mention of pregnancy. Without warning, my moment of panic came a few weeks later. Whatever smugness I felt evaporated when Laura's primary care physician called. I clicked on the speakerphone.

"Thanks," he offered, "for sending me your final summary of Laura's hospitalization. She was in and out so quickly I didn't even have time to visit her there. She and Stuart were in earlier today, and I reviewed the summary before their visit."

I sat up straight in my chair, fully attentive. Why was her doctor calling? I picked up the receiver, as I might pick up a rattlesnake, and pushed the button that turns off the speakerphone. My mouth was dry when I asked, "Is everything okay?"

"Sure," he comforted me, "but I was wondering, the hospital sent a copy of the record with the duplicate lab reports, and there was a positive pregnancy test."

A surge of nausea rose. At any other time, I would have praised the lab for being so efficient. "Oh what a tangled web…" Involuntarily, I glanced at my diploma on the wall. "A pregnancy test?" I managed to say. "Must be some mistake. That lab!" Then I added, my voice cracking just slightly, "You didn't say anything to Stuart, did you? You know he's had a vasectomy."

"Yeah, I knew that. That's why I'm calling. No, of course I didn't say anything. I guessed somebody goofed. Right?"

I became progressively more agitated as I realized that the information, the evidence of my duplicity, the false record although undisclosed, was out there forever, poised and waiting to strike. "Well," I said, grateful that no video was revealing the little beads of sweat on my forehead, "thanks for calling. Glad we got that straightened out."

"Yes," he affirmed. "I'm glad it's straightened out."

The problem with ethical dilemmas is the fallout—the uneasiness that remains after any choice is made. Inevitably, some evil is fostered or some good is left undone. Very often, the incident with Laura and Stuart intrudes into my thoughts. I know what Laura believes would have happened had I not arrogantly transgressed conventional morality. Nevertheless, I wonder whether I have harmed or helped Stuart by deceiving him. At the very least, it was disrespectful. Had I misjudged his ability to deal with a disruption in his marriage? Would his compulsive personality have forced him to separate from Laura as she feared, or could the two of them have become closer by working through this obstacle? Even for a perfectly centered person, I know that the wounds of infidelity heal slowly and the scars remain forever. Will the destructive secret that Laura must always hide distort her healing relationship with Stuart?

Aside from the moral dilemma, there's another consequence. I live every day with a disturbing question that darts unbidden, in and out of my consciousness. What will be the ending if someday, in anger or with trust and love, Laura reveals our conspiracy?

FAMILY

My receptionist buzzed me on the intercom. "Barbara Clark is on the phone. She wants to come in for a pregnancy test, but she got very upset when I told her we could do the test but we might not have time for a doctor visit today. It's Monday, you know. Your schedule's really full, but she says she can't wait for a visit later."

I shouldn't be surprised, I thought ruefully. This was the invariable something that shatters my good intentions to stay on schedule, but I felt it was particularly perverse for it to be the very first thing Monday morning.

"Put her through, Linda. Let's see what's up."

"What's the rush, Barbara?" I teased on the phone. "To find out if you're pregnant, all we need to do is wait."

Her voice was strained. You could almost see the tears running down her cheeks as she choked out, "Something awful has happened."

"What, what? Are you bleeding? Do you think you're miscarrying?" I asked, all jocularity gone in an instant.

"No, but I must see you now, and I—I can't talk on the phone," she stammered.

"Where are you, at home?"

"No, I'm here in town."

"Where's Paul?" I asked.

"He's home."

There was no use in trying to learn more over the phone. Panic was becoming audible in the atypical shrillness of Barbara's voice.

"Of course I'll see you," I said. "Come right over."

Barbara Craft was a pretty woman in her early twenties, out-doorsy and athletic, whom I had first met years before when she came for contraceptive advice. She was dating a man, she told me, who she had met at the Mountain Hiking Club. They had talked seriously of marriage, but he had some "old-fashioned" ideas about being financially stable before taking that step. He wanted to offer financial security to the woman he asked to be his wife. Barbara had a job she liked as a computer programmer for a local branch of a large national company, but Paul had just quit working for his father and was seeking to build his own condominium management business in a Colorado ski town.

Barbara had explained to me what Paul had revealed about his family—why he felt determined to get out from under his father's thumb and why he treasured independence so highly. Several years earlier, Tom, his older brother, had begun working for his father in the very lucrative family commercial land-development business, reluctantly deferring his deep-down desire to pursue journalism, his major in college. Soon Tom was making so much money he couldn't back away to follow his dream.

Paul abhorred how his parents had maneuvered Tom into their social circle, easing him into a lifestyle revolving around a country club with a dress code, tennis and golf tournaments, and admittedly worthy but stuffy charity balls. Paul despised the social circle of his parents, which also involved the consumption of much more alcohol than has been found useful for preventing heart disease. His greenish political leanings were precisely opposite those of his developer-father. Paul rebelled against the threat of a life managed by his parents, always in his father's shadow. He found pleasure in less-confining activities and had vastly different interests. Among many other things, he enjoyed skiing and hiking, and that's how he had met Barbara.

When Paul announced his intention to leave the family business, his father had become irate, overreacting as though taking the lid off long bottled-up anger at his rebellious son. Paul had never tried very hard to conceal his scorn for his older brother's subservience. His father was aware that he was being held in contempt by proxy, because it was his lifestyle that Paul so disdained.

"You were willing to use my money for college, weren't you," his father had sneered. "What's dirty about it now?" His mother's shoulders slumped as she settled further into her chair, subdued and letting the storm go on over her head. Over the years, she had adjusted—or, more accurately, had submitted—to being a well-cared-for possession of this domineering man. She had learned to ignore his unexplained absences and ostensibly solo business trips, but it had taken an increasing psychological and spiritual toll, and she had withdrawn more and more into herself.

Paul long before had learned his father had to be in charge of anything in which he partook—the golf tournaments, the kid's little league games, the barbecues, anything! When Paul, in grammar school, had failed to complete homework assignments, the teacher sent him home with a note suggesting a conference with his parents. His father had come blustering in to set the blame on anyone else, because his child could not be at fault. But he was not defending the child at all. Paul learned then that he, his brother, and his mother were merely subjects in his father's domain. His father was simply making clear that things and people in his dominion were extensions of him and were not to be trifled with. Paul knew he could never set his own course while he was working for his father. He was unwilling to yield to his father's dominance in exchange for easy money. Paul had sublimated the barely disguised antipathy toward his father into an irrepressible need to demonstrate he could be successful without his father's patronage.

And so he was! To establish himself, he had to move to a city that was a three-hour drive away. After a year, he had enough confidence in his business to ask Barbara to marry him. The first time Paul introduced Barbara to his parents, he was embarrassed by his father's slurred speech and ribald humor, brought on by two pre-dinner cocktails and most of the two bottles of wine they had with dinner. His parents were visibly annoyed that they had no influence on his choice of bride, but Barbara withstood the interrogation, and she was attractive, charming, well educated, and therefore acceptable. Barbara had a warm relationship with her parents and wanted to encourage a close family connection with Paul's as well. At Barbara's urging, Paul had maintained cordial relations with his parents, but his past experience with his father was an insurmountable barrier to true intimacy. So they had kept up contact by visiting occasionally for Sunday dinner (mostly for his mother's sake), and by allowing his father to pontificate without opposition, he avoided controversy.

After another year had passed, Barbara returned to my office and told me that she and Paul were ready to have a baby. We talked about good nutrition, continued exercise, and vitamin and mineral supplements, including the essential folic acid. Whenever the time came that she chose to discontinue using birth control pills, I advised her to use something else (like condoms) for a few months until her periods returned to the normal pre-pill pattern. She had never been a smoker. After we had finished a brief discussion of fetal alcohol syndrome (because we don't know exactly when it occurs in pregnancy or how much alcohol it takes to injure a fetus), she was quite willing to give up the occasional glass of wine she had with dinner or social events.

Now she was calling in a panic! What on earth could have gone wrong? On the last visit, we had spoken enthusiastically about a pregnancy. Was the marriage in trouble? What was she doing here in town when Paul was away in the distant town where they had moved when he started his business? Before Barbara arrived, I saw another patient; then the receptionist brought Barbara back the moment she came into the reception room. She was very agitated and in great distress.

The instant the door closed behind her, the tears she had dammed burst out, accompanied by wracking sobs. She had no makeup on, and her hair was in disarray—an altogether unusual appearance for this ordinarily poised woman. I said nothing, but handed her a fistful of tissues. Soon she controlled her sobs, although the tears continued to run down her cheeks as she related the events of the previous hours.

She and Paul had come to town Saturday to spend the weekend visiting at his parents' home. In retrospect, she recalled being taken aback by the more than affectionate greeting she had received from her father-in-law on their arrival. She attributed the slightly overheated paternal hug and kiss to the alcohol he had already consumed.

Saturday night, Paul's brother Tom and his wife joined them for dinner at the club. Paul had deliberately chosen a turtleneck shirt to wear, so the maitre d' could not foist a greasy necktie from the club's collection on him (as he always attempted to do when Paul wore his usual weekend open-collar shirt). Sunday night, Paul's parents served a pleasant dinner prepared at home. The bridge game that followed was somewhat trying because Paul's father again drank to excess. About ten-thirty, the phone rang, and Paul learned that a water pipe had burst in one of the condos he managed. Although the damage was only moderate, some of the units nevertheless were unusable, and he felt he had to return to organize the repair process.

Paul and Barbara had planned to stay at his parents' house Sunday night, in order to do some shopping Monday in the larger department stores of the city before they returned home. Paul suggested that Barbara stay over as planned. She could go on with the shopping trip, and he could return late in the afternoon to finish shopping with her and take her home. Worried that Paul would drive too fast in his anxiety about the tenants, Barbara waited up into the early morning hours until Paul completed the three-hour trip. After he had called her at about three in the morning, reassuring her that he had arrived safely, she went to bed in Paul's old room, where they usually stayed when they visited his parents overnight. Exhausted by worry and lack of rest, she quickly fell into a deep sleep.

More than half asleep, she felt someone who she thought was Paul slip into bed beside her—but that didn't make sense because he was away, wasn't he? Why was he away? Where was it that he had gone? He couldn't have returned yet, but—? Where was she now, if Paul had gone home? Her sense of time and place was fragmented—was she dreaming? Then a heavy hand clamped brutally across her mouth, and she awakened to the unthinkable as her father-in-law tore at her gown with his other hand and thrust his bulky body on her. The sweaty hand over her face muted her instinctive scream of outrage and astonishment. Before she was entirely awake, the rape had occurred. He rolled off, still holding his hand over her mouth, and whispered hoarsely in a fetid, alcohol-sodden breath, "Don't scream; I'm going." Then he was gone!

She lay there in bed, stunned. She reached down, hoping to find nothing, hoping she had had a horrible nightmare. But she saw the torn nightgown and felt the slimy wetness. Her fury surged as she thought of this brute, with his compulsion to possess, to control, to dominate. Suddenly, she was wide awake and trembling with anger. What could she do? Whom could she tell? Tears of frustration streamed down her face. Then, with alarm, she remembered that she had stopped her birth control pills so that she and Paul could have a baby. But she didn't want the spawn of his father—this predator, this thug! She went to the shower and washed and scoured and scrubbed, letting the hot water flush the outside of her body. She dressed, went to the phone, called a taxi, and called my office.

And there we were, trying to deal with the aftermath of this atrocity. As she related the story, she regained control of her tears and ended her account with questions. "What can I do? What should I do?"

I restrained my outrage—the angry urge to call the police instantly to arrest and to punish this depraved man. I forced myself to think, as a doctor usually needs to think, calmly and deliberately, about what had to be done immediately for Barbara.

"First," I said, "let's deal with the possibility of pregnancy. Where are you in your cycle?"

"Just about the middle."

"Then we have to use emergency contraception. Here are four contraceptive pills. These are the same thing they sell in the drugstore as a package." I pulled them from my desk drawer. "You take them within seventy-two hours of intercourse, and they'll prevent pregnancy. Take one right now and one more tonight; then tomorrow, take one in the morning and one at night. That's all you need, four of them."

"Okay."

"Now," I said, "I've got to examine you and collect evidence to report the rape to the police."

"Oh, no, no, no!" she gasped. "You can't—we can't do that."

"Don't do that?—But I must!—Don't you want that miserable lowlife to get what's coming to him?" I asked, flabbergasted at her dismay at what seemed so obvious to me.

"Paul would kill him," she blurted. "He hates him. I'd lose him; I'd lose Paul."

Whoa, I thought. This is not simple. Time out! I called the front desk and told the receptionist I had an emergency, to reschedule everyone that we possibly could. For the others, I'd be an hour behind. Barbara and I began to reexamine the situation.

"What are you thinking?" I asked her, still stunned by her response.

Barbara explained she could avoid virtually all contact with her father-in-law, and certainly need never be alone with him. It would not be hard to avoid overnight stays, or even social visits. Paul never initiated the visits. Barbara had suggested most of them, pushing the idea that family members ought to stay on good terms with each other.

Was this a crime that would be repeated? Certainly not for Barbara. She would never allow a situation to develop where it was even remotely possible. Barbara had been exhausted to the point of stupor and was therefore unresisting; she was sleeping in an isolated wing of the large house without Paul, trapped in a situation where the rapist knew she would not report the crime—circumstances unlikely ever to recur for her or anyone else.

But what about someone else? This attack, we concluded, was the act of a coward. This was a contemptible, opportunistic act by someone who would not dare to approach a woman who would or could resist; he was a coward who would not attack a woman who he knew would report the crime. It was a rare combination of circumstances that had allowed it to happen at all.

What would be the result if I reported it? There was no predicting what Paul might do. Barbara felt he would surely assault his father. As we spoke, Barbara's position became firmer. She would not consent to be examined; she would not make a complaint, nor be a willing witness. The consequences to everyone would be dreadful. The veneer of civility beneath which the family functioned was tenuous at best. This would tear the family apart. Paul's mother, for whom Paul felt compassion rather than disdain, always was on the verge of serious depression. She would have her remaining years shattered. Most of all, Barbara feared Paul's explosive reaction to the man, who in some sick and secret way had overcome his son's defiance. She could not risk that threat to her future with Paul. It far outweighed in her mind the burden of the terrible secret she must keep.

How would Barbara explain the awkwardness when she rejected all future social activity with the family? How would she be able to accommodate the rage that the memory of this barbarity would elicit in her? What would the pressure from the outrageous secret she was determined to keep from Paul do to their relationship? How would she explain to Paul that I had recommended counseling for her, alone? All this was wholly unpredictable, but this is often the case in medical practice. Decisions must be made with the best information available, which is often incomplete. Not even the wisest judge can augur the future. Ought I refrain from the public duty to report a felony to the police? I had to make my decision quickly. Barbara had made hers, and it appeared to be irrevocable.

Timing was significant. Delay in reporting a rape often makes the victim more the object of suspicion than the perpetrator. If we did not collect the evidence soon, it would be gone forever. If she would neither consent to an examination nor testify to the crime, then the case against the rapist would evaporate. Ought a criminal be exposed, no matter the consequences? Ought I bring charges regardless of my patient's wishes? How much risk was this man to the social order? Did my responsibility to my patient, and her wishes under these unique circumstances, overbalance my responsibility to the community?

Those were the questions we pondered first thing Monday morning.

Barbara tidied up in the office lounge, met Paul in the afternoon at the store, stifled her emotions, and went shopping.

I did not report the crime.

GENDER

For me, this story began in the 1960s, but for the patient, Vicki Chatham, it began much earlier, although she didn't know it at the time. Almost seventeen years after Vicki was born, I was making morning hospital rounds when the overhead pager called my name. When I picked up the phone at the nurse's station, the circulating nurse from an operating room gave me a message from the general surgeon operating there. He requested that I come to the operating room immediately to consult on a patient whose surgery was under way. His original plan had been to repair bilateral inguinal hernias for a young woman. This type of hernia results from weakness in the areas between the wide, flat muscles and the other tissues that support the lower area of the abdominal wall. Internal organs (such as the bowel) press against the thinned-out areas, stretching the tissue ahead of it. It ends up forming a structure that looks like an old-fashioned purse with a constricting purse string around the top. If the bowel squeezes through the narrow "purse string" and bulges out after it has gone through, it may be trapped. Then it would be called an "incarcerated hernia." If the trapped organ were bowel, it would be obstructed and in danger of rupture, spilling bacteria-laden bowel contents into the abdominal cavity. In the patient who I was called to see, there were two golfball–sized bulges just under her skin that, the surgeon told me, had caused her constant aching pain in the groin area.

Beneath the first incision, the surgeon had encountered a strange mass in the hernia canal, just above the labia. It didn't look like any hernia he had ever seen before. He had paged to ask me, as an experienced gynecologist, if I had ever seen this type of growth. Before I answered his question, I asked him if he had the menstrual history of the patient. He admitted he had instructed the intern to take that part of the history. To him, menstruation had not been relevant to what had appeared to be a straightforward case of inguinal hernias.

I picked up the chart and read the intern's note. He had written that this sixteen-year-old girl had not yet started menstruating. He noted she had told him she had never had sexual relations; therefore, there was no concern about pregnancy. I thought to myself that I must speak to him later and take the first opportunity to disenchant him of the notion that denial of sexual exposure unquestionably rules out pregnancy. In those days, there were no rapid pregnancy tests, so the intern relied on history and instinct, rather than risk the wrath of the surgeon by a last-minute postponement of the surgery until more tests could be run.

Based on this history, he assumed that the hymen was intact. This was an acceptable reason for him to dodge doing a pelvic examination for an adolescent female. The intern, not much older than the patient, had avoided this source of mutual uneasiness. I looked at the rest of the physical exam he had recorded and read, "normal post-pubertal breast development." Why had she not begun to menstruate? Vicki had completed breast development, which is usually a four-year process but is not completed until a patient has been menstruating a year or more. Menstruation, on average, begins about two-and-one-half years after breast development begins. This didn't add up. She should have started her periods.

One more clue remained to be sought. Before an operation in an area with body hair, it was usual then to shave the site and then wash it several times with bacteria-killing solutions. I asked the surgeon another question.

"Did you shave her when she was prepped for surgery?"

"No," he replied. "Didn't have to. I guess she does it herself. She didn't have any pubic hair when I checked the hernias pre-op."

I advised the surgeon to biopsy the mass in the hernia and send it to the lab for a frozen section that would provide an immediate diagnosis. Then I told him I expected the report would be "normal testicle."

He laughed and said, "You mean normal ovary, don't you?"

"No, I do mean normal testicle. I'll bet you're operating on a male," I replied.

ᕱ

Before we go further into Vicki's story, we need to spend some time unraveling the origin of gender. The first task is to understand basic physiology. We will have to go beyond the birds and the bees to explain, but we can stop short of molecular biology. In human reproduction, about 20 to 80 percent of fertilized eggs successfully implant in the wall of the womb before the end of the second week following fertilization. The rest do not survive and may be marked by a menstrual period delayed a few days.

The successful fertilized egg, by its second month, undergoes an exquisitely complex metamorphosis to continue from embryo to fetus. Demonstrating nature's remarkable economy, each embryo has the equipment to become male or female! Gender will depend on which chromosome combination the sperm has contributed—resulting in an XX for a female, an XY for a male. That combination will dictate the destiny of the gonad, determining whether it will be a female ovary or a male testis. It also points out the ignorance of many monarchs in the past who changed wives (sometimes through execution) when they did not produce a male heir to the throne. The gender is solely dependent on the husband's genetic contribution, and changing wives simply massaged masculine egos.

This is the critical point. For about eight weeks, all embryos have nonspecific genitals. A fetus (that is what they are called after eight weeks) will develop male genitals only under the stimulation of male hormones. A hormone is a chemical messenger circulating to all tissues through the bloodstream; it demands some response from those tissues that are equipped to receive its message. Without the positive influence of male hormones, the external genitals will always become female.

For a fetus to develop female genitals, it is the *absence* of male hormone—not the presence of female hormones—that is needed.

Male hormones are necessary for masculinization to occur. If they are not present, female external genitals will develop. Female hormones have no role in the fetal development of female genitals!

Now that you've gotten that straight, let me tell you how sometimes nature throws a monkey wrench into the usual machinery of genital development. Sometimes, the receptors for testosterone (a male hormone) are missing from the tissues that would have become the external male genitals. What does that mean to a potential male? Let me draw an analogy. There are all sorts of radio waves being transmitted all around you now, right? But if you don't have a radio, a receiver for the signals, you won't know anything about the radio programs. So, it sometimes happens that certain genetic messages are lost. Male external genital tissues that were supposed to receive testosterone messages in order to become a penis, for example, don't have a receiver. They are insensitive to testosterone. Because the tissues can't get the message, they don't masculinize, even though the fetus is an XY male and is developing testicles! The syndrome is called androgen insensitivity syndrome (AIS) because the tissues won't respond to male androgen. Androgen is the collective name for all the hormones that have masculinizing effects (testosterone is one of them).

Without the influence of testosterone, the fetus develops female external genitalia. But internally, the tissues that might have become ovaries, a uterus, and fallopian tubes in a female *do* have working receivers of a very different kind. They have receivers for signals that block female development. Their blocking receivers get the message from androgens that a male is being developed here, and their job is done. Those tissues that otherwise might have become a uterus, tubes, and ovaries are inhibited by the male hormones and fail to develop, partially or completely. The result is a chromosomal XY male with external female genitals (including the labia, clitoris, and some vagina), but the internal female genitals (uterus, tubes, and ovaries) are absent. The testicles formed in the abdomen may be found anywhere along the migration path to what would have been a scrotum. In this patient, the testicles had herniated into the canal that passes from inside the abdomen to the "scrotum," which in this situation had become the normal-appearing labia instead. The testicles hadn't completed their journey.

The short version of what happened to this patient is this: She had XY chromosomes, so testicles developed under their direction and produced androgens. The tissue that could have become either male or female external genitals did not have receptors for androgens, so they never got the message they were "supposed to be" male. Without that message, they automatically developed into female external organs—the labia, clitoris, and part of the vagina. The message from the male androgens "heard" by the potential female internal organs told them not to become female, so they retired from the field of operations. Consequently, no uterus, tubes, or ovaries, and very little vagina formed. You may be surprised to learn that testicles and ovaries each produce both male and female hormones in varying amounts. Breast tissue responded to the female hormones produced by the testicles. That's why she had normal breast development and a feminine body contour. Hair under the arms and in the pubic area results from androgen stimulation. Without receptors, virtually no sexual hair grows. She hadn't shaved—she simply had never grown pubic hair.

⌐

So let's go back to the operating room. There, the perplexed surgeon awaited an explanation for my seemingly absurd statement that this attractive young woman with feminine contours, including well-developed breasts and normal female external genitals, is a genetic male.

I carried the biopsy to the lab and watched the pathologist prepare the specimen. We looked at it through a teaching microscope that let us view it simultaneously. I explained my suspicions; the patient had "testicular feminization." That is what we called this condition in that era. We use the more appropriate term androgen insensitivity syndrome now that we understand the physiology better. The pathologist confirmed it was benign testicular tissue. It was a relief to have my diagnosis confirmed and even more of a relief that this patient was not one of the approximately 4 to 9 percent of people who have cancerous changes in undescended testicles. Cancer of the testicle in this type of patient is rare before puberty, but the hazard increases with age.

I returned to the operating room. I explained the situation to the surgeon, and he asked if I would accompany him when he spoke with the parents after the surgery. I agreed. I knew that many of these patients had a very short vagina despite the normal external appearance. The vagina is basically a tubular structure. Part of it comes from inside from the tissue that forms the internal female organs—the uterus, fallopian tubes, and ovaries. Part of it comes from outside from the external female organs—the labia and the clitoris. Then the two tube ends join together to form the whole vagina. Would it be ethical to do a pelvic exam while she was under anesthesia? We certainly hadn't gotten consent for it. Based on the balance of burdens and benefits, and the great value the information would have for future care, I decided to do the exam, provided I did not have to disrupt the hymen. I was able to do an exam without disturbing the hymen; there was almost none. There was a very shallow vagina within the labia. I felt no uterus or ovaries. I didn't expect to find them. I knew the patient would be sterile. Something would have to be done if, despite sterility, she desired a deeper, functioning vagina for sexual intimacy.

I also urged the surgeon to remove the testicles in the hernias. If the patient hadn't reached puberty, that might not have been done until the female hormones from the testicles could do what they had already achieved for her. That is, pubertal changes had already occurred; oral female hormones would be available to maintain normal breasts and other feminine contours even if the unusual source of estrogen for Vicki, the testicles, were removed. Taking oral female hormones was the trade-off in order to reduce the risk of future testicular cancer by removing the testicles. We could have taken the time to go to the waiting room to speak with the parents about removing the testicles as the hernias were repaired. We rejected that idea because the time that would have been required would have unnecessarily prolonged anesthesia. We were taking some legal and ethical risks because we truly believed, on balance, they were in the patient's interest.

With the surgery completed, other problems presented. We quickly decided that we would explain all of this confusing information to the parents as often and completely as necessary until they understood it all. Our dilemma was deciding what ought we counsel the parents to say to their daughter. How much of this information ought be told to the patient? What impact would the knowledge of a masculine chromosome configuration and the presence of testicles have on her self-image, combined with the knowledge that her vagina was not normal and she was sterile? What ought we explain to her, and when would be the best time to speak about her sterility?

⌐

Even with the advantage of hindsight, not all of these answers are clear. Some things we said and did, in all probability, we would do differently today. Things change. We all know that, but we sometimes fail to realize how fast they can change. Back in the dark ages of the 1960s, when this story took place, there were no CT-scans or MRIs. Now, these marvels of imaging let a doctor see the soft tissues, the inner organs, of a patient almost as well as they could by looking inside through an incision. Even the less-revealing ultrasound was in its infancy. X-rays are of very little value for revealing the soft-tissue details of the female organs.

Today, if we need to see what's going on in the pelvis and abdomen of a shy adolescent, we can use these noninvasive tools. But before these devices existed, the details of the internal anatomy of a young woman were a mystery. The fine points would remain obscure unless a frightened patient, a reluctant doctor, and anxious parents were willing to undertake an invasive surgical procedure.

Some variant of AIS occurs in one in twenty thousand births. Outside of medical referral centers, few pediatricians or obstetrician-gynecologists have seen such cases. It was unlikely that surgeons would see such patients except those with hernias, an even smaller number of cases per professional lifetime. Today, in keeping with a wonderful trend in medical coping, there are support groups for such patients, with contact information and good explanations to be found on the Internet by searching for androgen insensitivity syndrome or intersex support groups.[3] There were no such support entities in the early sixties. Then the method of managing this was secrecy, as if the condition were something to be ashamed of, and patients felt very isolated. More treatment options are now available for the undersized vagina; sometimes surgery can be avoided. Hormone treatment is essential to ameliorate the hazard of bone weakness, the same osteoporosis that occurs in the postmenopausal woman without estrogen. Because of all we have learned over four-plus decades, withholding information would be considered unethical today. There are many intermediate variations of intersexuality, and in cases of truly ambiguous genitals, current recommendations are to await the patient's maturity and allow the completely informed patient to determine whether they wish to maintain or alter their body configuration. In the partial androgen insensitivity syndrome, different levels of androgen effects may lead to gender ambiguity. Patients may feel attraction to either or both males and females. That doesn't appear to be a problem in the complete androgen insensitivity syndrome, which was the case for Vicki.

We didn't have much of this knowledge or most of these tools when this patient was first seen. In hindsight, we made mistakes. Her parents and I decided to avoid telling her about the XY chromosomes and the testicles that were removed. We based our ethical reasoning on a system called "consequentialism." Prophets and philosophers have been struggling for thousands of years to distinguish good from bad, right from wrong. The problems that are called dilemmas are especially trying. Dilemmas have the disturbing characteristic that no matter which choice is made, some evil will result or some good will be left undone. There is always leftover uneasiness, some "moral fallout," because it's impossible to reach a perfect solution.

Many of today's arguments and dilemmas begin with fundamental differences. Does absolute authority reside in ancient sources of moral direction, or must there be modifications because of changes in the times and manners? You may recognize this as the debate about moral absolutism versus moral relativism.

When most people have to make a decision about everyday matters, they usually try to predict the outcome and choose the alternative that promises the best result for them. That idea of speculating upon the consequences of decisions is at the heart of the ethical system for decision making called consequentialism (or utilitarianism). In order to consider it an ethical system for making societal choices, people would have to include more than themselves in the balance sheet. They would have to consider what would produce the most value over disvalue for everyone, not just for themselves. This approach is often abbreviated, "the greatest good for the greatest number."

Because it is impossible always to predict consequences, another system called deontology is used that determines the ethical choice provided certain rules are followed. Such imperatives include keeping promises, never lying or deceiving, never exploiting persons, and always acting in a way that you would want others to always act.

You can easily see where conflicts may arise between these two systems. You can conjure up a scenario, I'm sure, when a lie under special circumstances would clearly bring about a better outcome for everyone. That would be the right thing to do because it was the good thing to do (for a consequentialist). But a deontologist, who believes you have rules to follow regardless of consequences, would mark your behavior as unethical.

So, a deontologist would have told us to tell the truth from the beginning. As consequentialists, we thought it would be better not to confuse or upset the young woman with the unusual facts of her gender. Dealing with sterility and possibly the need for some vaginal reconfiguration, we felt, was trauma enough without adding gender identity questions as well. In retrospect, we realize how we paternalistically decided that it was better for Vicki to have "female *problems*" than to have questions about *being* female.

Today, patients with complete androgen insensitivity syndrome such as Vicki's—clearly very female in mind and body—might think it absurd for a doctor to raise a question about their gender or suggest that it was a question of preference rather than it being patently obvious. "Of course I am female! Chromosomes be damned!" most would declare.

But other cases have been reported in which female gender assignment was made at birth and surgical alterations were made to conform. Despite social pressures, there came a time when this uneasy patient could no longer deny that a spurious gender had been assigned and critical life changes were necessary for him. They were vastly complicated by the too early commitment to gender. But those are other stories and not Vicki's.

VICKIE'S PARENTS

When we arrived in the waiting area, we were pleased to see both parents sitting together chatting. So often, a father will continue to work while Mom waits alone, then calls him to say everything is all right. The first thing the surgeon said to Vicki's parents was that she was fine and there were no problems with the hernia repairs. They expressed relief and thanks. He then introduced me as a gynecologist with whom he had consulted because of the unusual structures that were part of the hernia. He said that I would explain. They turned to me.

"Vicki doesn't have cancer or any other life-threatening condition," was the first thing I said. "Lets go to that little room over there where we can talk about it in private."

They came with me to a small consulting room, and we sat down across from each other.

"We found some things out that are going to be important to Vicki's future, but I truly believe things will turn out okay. There are problems, but we can deal with them. I guess there is no easy way to say this, but the biggest problem is, unfortunately, Vicki will not be able to have children. It had nothing to do with the operation. It was a condition she was born with."

Mrs. Chatham's face darkened. "Was it something I did when I was pregnant with her?"

Mr. Chatham put his hand on Mrs. Chatham's arm in a comforting gesture. His movement was reassuring to me also because it gave me a feeling that this was a solid family and that would make a hard task somewhat easier.

"Oh, absolutely not," I assured her. "Nothing you did could have prevented it. This may be something that passed down in your family. About two-thirds of cases are inherited, and one third just happens during pregnancy—no one knows why. You might be a carrier of the gene, but even if you knew, there's nothing you could have done about it. Does Vicki have sisters?"

"No."

"And you've stopped menstruating?" I asked.

"Yes."

"Then there aren't going to be more babies, so there'll be no new problems from this."

"What do we need to do? What should we tell Vicki?" she asked.

"Well, I'm sure you know Vicki hasn't been sexually active."

"Of course she hasn't," her mother responded, only mildly indignant. "She's only sixteen. She's had a few dates—but only with nice boys, though."

"Vickie has an unusual problem that causes her to be infertile," I explained. "Part of this condition is a problem with the vagina," I said. "It has not developed completely and it is not deep enough for sexual intercourse."

"Oh, my," Mrs. Chatham responded, then, "What can we do," she asked weeping silently. "She can't have a normal life, that way."

"We can fix the vagina. She can have a normal life except she won't be able to become pregnant. You know, 15 percent of all women can't have children. But she is normal in all other respects, and adoption is always an option, if she and a future husband want kids."

Again, she asked, "Why did this happen? If it isn't something I did, what caused it?"

"Well, it's a complicated story that's all about genetics and hormones," I replied, "but I'd like to explain it, and you feel free to interrupt and ask questions if I don't make it clear. And, while we're at it, keep in mind how much of this we ought to explain to Vicki." I then carefully related the mechanism for genital formation to Vicki's parents and how it came to affect her. They asked me to repeat frequently, but they appeared to understand it sufficiently. I was glad they did not hesitate to agree that we had done the right thing by removing the testicles and, with that, the cancer risk. They thought that it would only cause unnecessary anxiety for Vicki if we spoke about testicles and raised the issue of male chromosome configuration. We agreed simply to avoid that while we confronted the problem of sterility and the influence on sexual intimacy of vaginal depth.

"Can we be in the room when you tell Vicki about it?" Mr. Chatham asked.

"How do you think Vicki would feel when I begin discussing her sexual activity?"

"We've always been completely open with her, and discussions about sexuality have been easy, even with her father," Mrs. Chatham replied. "But maybe we should let Vicki decide whether she wants us there when you talk about sexual activity—I mean about fixing the vagina and things."

"Well, I'll certainly tell her what I've explained to you except what we've agreed to skip over, and we'll see if she wants to talk it over with you or with all of us together. I'm sure you'll think of more questions—and also you should feel free to speak with other doctors. It would probably be wise to have Vicki consult with a psychiatrist because, no matter how well adjusted anyone might be, this is an awful lot to absorb at once, and she's going to need help to adjust to the whole idea. With your permission, I'm going to ask one who has experience with adolescents to see her while she's still in the hospital. Okay?"

꙳

After I returned to my office, I began to consider how to explain things to Vicki. I remembered my first contact with the AIS and resolved that what I had observed in medical school was not going to be repeated with her. There, three residents had assembled with the attending gynecologist to examine a patient with the same condition. I'm sure this made her feel freakish, and I've regretted it ever since. Of course, students must learn, as I did at the time. But at the very least, the patient must be a truly willing participant, not pressured into accepting the role of an exhibit. Certainly, no more than one student ought accompany the teacher. The surgical intern and the resident who scrubbed on Vicki's operation had learned the lesson about the possibilities for "hernia" in a young woman without causing embarrassment. Photographs without identifying features would suffice to teach this condition without adding to the patient's disquiet.

SPEAKING WITH VICKIE

I was able to make evening rounds at the hospital early, so I could begin explaining the findings to Vicki before she had a chance to question the nurses or her parents. I thought they might feel they couldn't explain it well to her and, by deferring the discussion, would appear evasive. That would set the wrong tone for managing her care.

"Hello, Vicki. I'm Dr. Abrams. I was there at your surgery, and I've already met your parents."

Vicki looked at me quizzically. She appeared to have recovered from the anesthesia, thinking clearly enough to say, "I thought Dr. Francis was the one who was going to operate on me."

"Of course, and he did operate and he repaired the hernias. I'm sure he'll be making rounds soon, and he'll be pleased to see how nicely you're recovering. I'm a gynecologist, and he called me in because he found some things that he felt someone in my specialty could manage better because we have more experience in that field."

"Oh, and what was that?" I thought that perhaps she was feigning casualness as a defensive mechanism, but she responded in a no-nonsense tone that encouraged me to believe this was a self-possessed young woman.

"First, let me assure you that there isn't anything that is a threat to your life and health. That's certain, but I don't know any easy way to tell you this and I don't know how important it will be for you, but we found you will not be able to become pregnant and have children."

There was silence. Vicki frowned and turned to her parents and asked, "Did he tell you this already?" They nodded. "Why—why can't I have children?" she asked, turning to me. "What's wrong with me?"

"Most of the time when this happens, it's a genetic condition that you inherit. Less often, it isn't inherited; we just don't know why it happens. There's no way to prevent it, and there's no way anyone could have known about it in advance. But let me tell you it's nothing your parents did or anything you did that caused it. Unfortunately, there isn't any way to treat it, either. I mean, there's no way to make you fertile."

Again, silence as she absorbed the information, then tears. Her mother got up and embraced her, crying silently as her father moved to hold her hand. I thought, *That's enough for one day; some time alone with her parents would be appropriate.* After a moment, I said, "I'm going to see some other patients, then come back to talk more and answer questions—mostly to set up a time to talk tomorrow, after you've had some time to think about it."

In those days, hernia was an in-patient procedure, not day surgery as is usual now—when patients are discharged the same day that surgery is performed. Then, patients stayed at least overnight and often another day for recuperation. I was glad I would have time to speak at length with Vicki before she went home.

The next morning, Vicki was up, dressed, and sitting on the edge of her bed, her feet dangling and her small suitcase on the floor when I came in. I hadn't been able to contact the psychiatrist yet, and it didn't look as if Vicki wanted to wait in the hospital for any consultation.

"Looks like you may be anxious to get out of here," I observed with a smile. "You don't seem to have much pain from the operation, do you?"

"No," she said. "Do I have to wait for Dr. Francis?"

"It would be better. He'll want to give you some instructions about taking care of the incision and what activity is okay and stuff."

"You said you wanted to talk to me about what's wrong. Can we do that now, or do I have to come to your office?"

I knew that in the long run, the psychological problems were more difficult to manage than the physiological ones, so I said, "Well, both, really. There are some medications you'll need to take, and I'd like to supervise that, and I'd like to recommend some counseling. No matter how well adjusted a person is, the kind of information I've given you—and there's some more explanation we can talk about now—it's hard to take. Everyone needs someone with experience to talk about it with and to help them come to terms with it."

This time, the higher-pitched voice registered the alarm that had been just under the surface all along. "What else is there? There's more?"

"Well, yes. Let me explain. I want to tell you again, there's nothing life- or health-threatening about this. The problem you have is hormonal. You remember I told you yesterday that you wouldn't be able to have children. I didn't go into details then. The reason you can't have children is because the hormones weren't working right when you were in your mom's uterus. You've probably noticed that almost all your classmates have begun to menstruate already. Were you curious about that?"

"Yes. I was going to wait for my next birthday to talk to mom about that. But I've got breasts and everything." Then, hesitating for a moment, she cocked her head and looked hard at me. "You're a GYN, so I can be honest with you, can't I? No sense in being embarrassed. Right?"

"Sure."

"Well, I've masturbated, so I wasn't worried."

I confess I was startled by her matter-of-fact declaration, but I think it didn't show, and I maintained an air of concerned detachment. *In fact,* I quickly reflected to myself, *that's going to make this much easier than I thought it would be.*

"Good," I said. "That shows you can have normal sexual response despite some changes internally." I picked up where I had left off with the topic of menstruation. "You see, you haven't menstruated, and you can't become pregnant because your uterus and ovaries didn't develop internally and your vagina didn't grow as deep as it should have. You're going to need to take hormones to keep your figure. And estrogens do other very important things, too, like keeping your bones strong."

"So I'll be taking hormones forever?"

"Pretty much. About the vagina, now. Your parents wanted to know if you wanted them to be here when we talked about all this. Do you?"

"Well, we're talking about it now, so let's finish up and I'll tell them what we talked about. They're pretty open, and we talk a lot."

"Let's talk a little anatomy first. Ordinarily, the vagina is a tube that connects at the top with the opening to the uterus, the cervix."

"We learned all that."

"Okay. Because the internal organs didn't develop, the vagina is not as long as most."

"So what does that mean? I'm not ready for sex anyway."

"Someday, in all likelihood, you're going to be. Then you may find out it isn't deep enough to have intercourse. There are several ways to fix that, if you want to. I can make it deeper surgically, but it's not always necessary to do that. First of all, when you have sexual relations, you may find out it is deep enough already. Depends a little on your husband. Just having sex will deepen it, too. Second, when you're ready to have sexual relations, if you need to, you can deepen it using some dilators. But you have to use them every day for a while. I can teach you how, and just pressing them in will deepen the vagina in a month or two with very little discomfort. But in the event these things don't work, I can make a deeper vagina surgically. We'll consider that when you're really ready for sexual intimacy. The bottom line is, I know women with this problem who have normal sex lives and normal marriages, and some have adopted children."

"Wow, that's a lot to think about. Do you have any more surprises for me? I don't need any more. You've told me everything now?"

"No more surprises." I dodged the question with a little twinge of conscience because obviously, I hadn't told her *everything*—for her own good, I thought. "Let's make an appointment in my office. Bring your parents if you want to. I'll have an appointment lined up with a psychiatrist who's familiar with this, and I think it's really important to see her. We'll plan on starting hormones then and reviewing everything. Now, wait for Dr. Francis to discharge you, and I'll see you in a week or so."

I believe I made Vicki's life a little easier by skipping talk of testicles and XX/XY chromosomes. Today, it would be considered poor practice to withhold information. What's more, it would be virtually impossible. The patient would be on the Internet in no time and know more about her condition than many doctors. But that kind of easy access to medical information didn't become available until Vicki was in her forties.

As society opened up, began to explore sexuality, and shed taboos along with unnecessary secrecy, I learned a lot about the pitfalls of paternalism and the merits of patient autonomy. However, Vicki never reexamined the etiology of her genital configuration. She and I got to know each other well. We created a functioning vagina without resorting to surgery, using dilators. She maintained a therapeutic relationship with her psychiatrist, which turned out to be decisive as she dealt—successfully— with anxiety about sexual inadequacy. There were ups and downs while she was dating. During her mid-twenties, a crisis occurred when a man with whom she had become quite serious broke off the relationship when he learned she couldn't have children of her own. With support from her friends, her parents, the psychiatrist, and me, she overcame that setback. Then she went on to meet other men, and, thirty-one years later when I retired from practice, she provided me with an old-fashioned Hollywood ending. As we said good-bye, we admired together the series of photographs that I had clipped into her record over the years. Just inside the chart's back cover was a picture of Vicki, her husband, and their two adopted daughters.

CONFIDENTIALITY

Whatever I see or hear, professionally or privately,
which ought not to be divulged, I will keep secret and tell no one.
—Hippocratic Oath

"Lots of people feel that when you've reached a certain age, it's your own business whether you're having sexual intercourse or not. Most of the time, only two people are concerned. But if you become pregnant, it becomes everybody's business. That's a pretty hard secret to keep, and, at your age, it affects many people—your parents, at the very least, for example."

I was delivering this message to seventeen-year-old Susan Forland, whose mother had brought her to see me "for a checkup." Susan had just answered my question about whether she had been sexually active—a question I sandwiched between bladder functions and bowel activity as I reviewed all the body's systems with her before doing a physical examination. The advantage of placing the question exactly there was twofold. First, it fell into place casually along with other queries about normal body functions, so it didn't feel like prying. Second, it was asked so matter-of-factly that the adolescent, ordinarily reluctant to discuss this loaded subject, answered it before she had a chance to consider whether she should admit to a sometimes-taboo activity.

"Yes," she said. "I'm pretty sure that's why Mom brought me."

"For birth control?"

"Yes."

"So you've told her?"

"Not exactly, but she knows I've been going steady with Roger since we were sophomores, and we stay home alone to babysit my little sister. We've talked about sex—Mom and I—and I think she's cool with it."

"So, why haven't you asked her flat out if you should take the pill or something?"

"I don't know."

"Well, should we ask her now, after I've examined you and figured out what would be best?"

"Yes, then it will all be out in the open, but Dad will be pissed. Oops! Is it okay to say that?"

Susan had made it much easier for me, now that she was willing to involve her mother in the consultation. It's difficult to prescribe contraception for a young woman who you think may not have explored the implications of sexual activity. In that case, without knowing the family's attitudes and values, I must act in loco parentis. Doctors may take much more responsibility on their shoulders, because doctors are often witness to the impulsive behavior of adolescents and the power of hormones. It's better to know she has delved into the significance of sexual intimacy with someone she trusts who is presumably more experienced than she is in human relations.

Yet for less-well-functioning families, it becomes necessary for the doctor to do much more weighing and balancing of possible consequences when the parents are not privy to the consultations. Reliable research has shown that virtually all young, single people who come in for contraception have already had intercourse, often more than once. Refusing to provide birth control and substituting instead a lecture extolling the virtues of abstinence is rarely contraceptive. When a discussion with a young woman reveals that abstinence is unlikely, it is hard to refuse contraception, knowing that unwanted pregnancy would be the most likely outcome.

"Have you used anything so far?"

"Most of the time, we've used condoms, but I'd really like the pill because I'm in control of that; and besides, I've heard it really helps the cramps."

Of course, we did much more talking that day about birth control. When we came to sexually transmitted diseases, Susan said that wouldn't be a problem because neither her boyfriend, who was a high school classmate, nor she would be seeing anyone else. "In a few years," she said, "we'll be getting married." We invited her mother in after the exam. When our discussion was over, Susan left with low-dose oral contraceptives and a follow-up appointment.

૮

That was my first visit with Susan. Over the years, there were many more. Susan came in every year for her pap smear and exam, even after she went off to college. Susan's heartbreak came when she and her boyfriend went away to different colleges, pledging eternal fidelity. At their first Christmas break, he brought home a gift of chlamydia. Chlamydia, for those who haven't heard of it, is not a bouquet of tropical flowers as the exotic name might suggest. It is the most common sexually transmitted disease.

A few weeks later, after they had both returned to school, she wrote and told him that their vacation-time unprotected intercourse had had unexpected results. She told me she deliberately hadn't written in her letter exactly what the "unexpected result" was, so "he could stew for a while." He telephoned her in a panic, expecting that she was "expecting." On the telephone, she advised him that she had become psychic in the last three weeks. Now, she told him, she could foretell their future. He'd see a doctor soon, she predicted, and also, he'd never see her again. She then proceeded to flagellate him with reference to his character using vocabulary from Chaucer, demonstrating for skeptics the value of an education in the classics. And that ended her first love affair, with her self-esteem damaged but no lasting physical injury.

When I treated her for chlamydia, she swore she would never have sex again until she was engaged to be married. I didn't wish to sound unsympathetic when I advised her I would not think ill of her should she request contraception even before she wore a diamond ring. She sheepishly but wisely returned for contraception again the following summer, and I extolled the virtues of barrier methods such as condoms, perhaps with the pill as well. The first protected against sexually transmitted diseases; the second against unwanted pregnancy. As I warned her, "There's a lot of both of them going around. Besides, it's like using a belt *and* suspenders for security—if one failed, there'd be a backup."

Susan was graduated with honors and found a job with the local newspaper as a reporter; she soon had achieved sufficient experience and expertise to merit frequent bylines. We had less eventful annual visits, and she shared her adventures—social and occupational—with me. Susan traversed the social scene with occasional liaisons just like many bright, independent young women of the late seventies and early eighties. She assured me, when I spoke of the dangers of casual sex, that she really wasn't intimate with just anyone. Rather, it was an acceptable behavior among her peers to test an alliance to rule out sexual incompatibility before a relationship deepened. I thought to myself that I wasn't with it—this generation. We old fuddy-duddies considered that the reverse order of activity was better, friendship before sex. At least we gave lip service to that idea. But the more I thought about it, the less sure I became that it really worked that way.

꙳

Something else was happening in the eighties that no one would have predicted would have any imaginable connection to Susan. A rare form of cancer, Kaposi's sarcoma, had manifested itself as an uncommon skin lesion in a cluster of eight young men in New York City. Shortly thereafter, an observant technician alerted the Centers for Disease Control (CDC) in Atlanta that there had been an unusual number of requests for a drug used primarily for a rare type of infection, *Pneumocystis carinii* pneumonia. The CDC published a report of a cluster of five men in Los Angeles with this unusual lung disease without explaining the source. In July 1981, the observation that these illnesses were all in homosexual men gave rise to the idea that it was a sexually transmitted disease confined solely to homosexuals.

By the end of the year, when intravenous drug users were found to be afflicted with immunodeficiency disease, that idea was abandoned, but very slowly. One of the early names persisted, "GRID"— gay-related immune deficiency. Then it appeared in a number of Haitians, so the CDC placed that entire citizenry in the high-risk category. After four years, it had become apparent that contaminated needles and heterosexual contact were significant factors, and the CDC removed Haitians from their list of high-risk groups. This action was followed by reports of infection in hemophiliacs who received large amounts of transfused blood derivatives. A hemophiliac could receive products derived from as many as five thousand different donated units of blood. Coupled with the widely reported death of a twenty-month-old infant who also had been transfused, the appearance in diverse groups began to divert attention from gay men and toward fear of blood transfusions. It also became apparent as reports came in from Europe that the disease, which was ultimately named AIDS (Acquired Immunodeficiency Disease), was not confined to the United States. What appeared to be a new plague was reported from Africa and was called "slim disease," because the patients appeared to waste away. Information accumulated showing that heterosexual women also were infected.

No causative agent had yet been identified, nor was it known precisely how it spread. People feared contagion by casual contact. Police in San Francisco were supplied with masks and gloves to be used when they were involved with persons who might be carriers. In the United Kingdom, people who were considered susceptible were asked to not donate blood. In 1983, the French Pasteur Institute lab isolated a virus as a probable cause and sent a specimen to the U.S. National Cancer Institute (NCI). A year later, the NCI reported they had isolated the virus that caused AIDS. Researchers disputed whether it was the same as the French isolate. Credit for the discovery was debated, but as you may have guessed, all the litigation revolved around the money to be derived from the patents on the AIDS diagnostic test. The international dispute was settled a few years later with an agreement to share profits.

The political and civil liberty aspects of the disease were always smoldering, but protests over the closure of gay bathhouses and private sex clubs in San Francisco occupied the headlines in 1984. When a blood test was patented in 1985, new ethical issues were encountered. Confidentiality was crucial, as ignorance led to fear, and fear led to abominable behavior across the country. Ryan White, a thirteen-year-old hemophiliac who had contracted AIDS from a blood transfusion, was barred from school. New anxieties arose when it was reported that an infant had been infected through breast-feeding.

The federal judiciary became involved because of federal antidiscrimination law when a nurse was dismissed from a hospital because he had AIDS. But the executive branch was less sympathetic. It wasn't until 1985 that President Reagan mentioned AIDS publicly, and it did not help relieve fears when he responded to a question by the press as to whether he would (if his children were younger) send them to a school where a child had AIDS.

Reagan replied, "It is true that some medical sources had said that this cannot be communicated in any way other than the ones we already know and which would not involve a child being in the school. And yet medicine has not come forth unequivocally and said, 'This we know for a fact, that it is safe.' And until they do, I think we just have to do the best we can with this problem. I can understand both sides of it."

That was also the year that the drug AZT (azidothymidine) was tested, one of many that were tried. It was not a new drug. It had been tested in the sixties as an anticancer drug, but it didn't work. Two groups of patients were in the trial. One group received the drug; the other received a placebo. After six months, there were nineteen deaths in the placebo group and only one in the group treated with AZT. The trial was stopped because it would have been unethical to continue using placebos when the actual medicine was apparently effective, at least in the testing period.

Also during this period, three boys from the Ray family who were hemophiliacs had contracted AIDS from blood products. In 1986, the boys were banned from their Florida schools. The family moved to Alabama, and again the children were not permitted to enroll in school. Petitions and protests reflected community anger and fear. After numerous anonymous threats, their house was burned down. It took many years and four pivotal district and Supreme Court cases before children with AIDS were allowed to go to school, based primarily on the federal Americans with Disabilities Act.[4]

Numerous methods for containing the disease were advanced by politicians and the public, including quarantine or detention camps that would provide facilities for entire families if they were related to the AIDS victim. Others suggested mandatory universal testing and wide publication of the names of all people testing positive. After several patients of a single dentist in Florida were infected, a powerful movement began to pass a federal law mandating that all health care workers be tested—doctors, dentists, and any others who worked directly with patients. The value of such testing would be questionable as a preventive measure, because it took up to six months after contact before an individual would turn seropositive; that is, showing a positive test result. If surgeons were tested daily, they would soon become too anemic to operate.

The leadership of the United Kingdom was more sympathetic and reassuring to the public. When Princess Diana opened an AIDS hospital in England, she shook hands with patients after removing her gloves. The United Kingdom also initiated a syringe exchange program so addicts would not spread the disease with contaminated needles. This suggestion was met with much opposition in the United States because it was seen as encouraging drug use. Some local programs were begun, but Congress prohibited the use of federal funds for such programs.

In the United States, states passed varying laws about reporting the results of AIDS tests. The difference between a positive test for the virus and the actual symptomatic disease was not clear, especially regarding the potential for infecting others. Only gradually and begrudgingly did people begin to accept that only sustained exposure to body fluids—primarily blood products, semen, and vaginal exudates—carried significant risk. Unfounded fear of shared eating utensils, towels, tears, and saliva continue to persist.

Informed consent was stressed, so persons could not be tested without their knowledge. Exceptions were made for exposed health care workers and law-enforcement personnel, and also for criminals who might have exposed victims. Counseling before testing and confidentiality after it were requested. After treatment methods were found in the late 1980s, AIDS turned from a brief and fatal disease to a so-far incurable but manageable chronic disease. Before that turnaround, high-risk persons found the hazards of discrimination more threatening than the disease, because no good treatment was offered. When somewhat effective treatment was available, high-risk persons had reason to find out so treatment could be started. But would their disease status remain confidential? The debate about whether anonymous testing should be allowed began. Would persons with the disease warn their contacts? Could employers, landlords, and insurance companies learn results that would lead to discrimination if testing were not anonymous? Schools and hospitals had already shown their disposition toward AIDS victims. What should be revealed in the interest of public health as opposed to individual interests?

Colorado was the first state to make a report by name mandatory for those testing positive for HIV (Human Immunodeficiency Virus). All laboratories where tests were done had strict confidentiality rules. They could report only to the ordering physician and the public health department. This policy did take much of the onus off doctors. Doctors could not give the information to any contacts of patients who tested positive, but they did have to report to the department of public health, which then had the responsibility to determine contacts and warn those they knew of. And that's how we come back to Susan.

~

If Susan's contact had been tested later, after anonymous testing was permitted in Colorado, we would probably never have learned of her risk. She still had the feeling that "nice" people didn't have to worry about AIDS. She didn't believe her "crowd" included intravenous drug users, although she knew that many smoked pot—and maybe some might have snorted cocaine on rare occasions. She hadn't used drugs, nor did she wish to. Obviously, anyone with whom she was intimate manifestly liked women. It never entered her mind that a man to whom she was physically attracted could be bisexual.

Susan had been dating a coworker at the newspaper office for over a year when I saw her for her GYN checkup. Testing for the virus had become available. People had become cautious. It had not been unusual for some of my single, sexually active patients to arrange for simultaneous testing with their prospective partner before they became intimate. Indeed, Susan and her partner, Tim, had done this about a year before, and she did not wish to repeat the test at her annual visit. She explained that she feared her insurance company would learn of the test through the coding of her bill and inquire why she felt at risk. The bill would also pass through the administrative office of her new employer. That might be prejudicial. Many patients were concerned about confidentiality related to health insurance coverage and their employers. Refusal of coverage and employment bias was being actively litigated.

I explained that the tests were confidential, but that did not assuage Susan's concern. She told me that she and Tim had been speaking seriously about marriage. They had been living together for about six months, and, except for Tim's occasional trips to visit his parents in Sausalito, they spent all their spare time together. I didn't urge testing, knowing they had done it about a year before, and she told me she had been in a monogamous relationship since. About a month later, I was made painfully conscious of this decision by a phone call from an internist with whom I "shared" several patients.

"Hi, Fred," he greeted me. "I think you take care of Susan Forland. Right?"

"For about eight or ten years. Is she seeing you for something? I just did a GYN checkup last month."

"No, she isn't my patient, but her fiancé is."

"Oh, fiancé? Did they make it official? She told me she was getting serious about Tim…'Somebody'. I forgot his last name."

"Well, he's the one who told me about her, and he said 'fiancé.' He said he was going to be married, and I asked him who the lucky lady was."

"Okay, so what about Susan?"

"Well, there's something Susan needs to know, and I can't tell her. In fact, I can't even tell you, but I've got to."

"What? What do you mean?"

"Let's say I'm going to break a state law, and when I do, I'd like to feel you're not going to tell anybody—anyone at all, including Susan—where you got this information. Because she's going to ask, you know. And you've got to figure out some way to tell her without involving me."

"Okay, okay. What's so mysterious that I can't tell anyone?"

"Well, in a word, Tim tests positive for HIV."

I was dumbfounded. Susan and Tim had been tested within the year. At least, I knew with certainty that Susan had been tested, because I had ordered the test and had seen the result. I assumed Susan had seen Tim's results, too, but I hadn't asked her. She simply had told me they both were going to be tested. I paused long enough for the doctor on the phone to ask, "Fred, are you there?"

"Yes, I'm here, but it doesn't figure."

"What doesn't figure?"

"Tell me," I asked, "is this the first time you've tested Tim?"

"No, I tested him a year ago when he said he and Susan soon were going to be living together and they both were going to be tested. That's when he told me you were her doctor and were going to do the test on her."

"Yes, that's when I had Susan checked, and she was negative, and I assume Tim was negative too, right?"

"Yes."

"So he converted from negative to positive over the year?"

"Well, I'm getting into this deeper and deeper telling you this, but the reason he asked me to test him again is because he's been stopping over in a bathhouse in San Francisco when he visits his parents in Sausalito."

"Wow! Is he going to tell Susan?"

"That's the problem. He knows I have to notify public health—the lab will, anyway—but he knows about doctor-patient confidentiality and that I can't tell anybody. And he told me he's not going to tell them about contacts outside of San Francisco. It's still voluntary, you know. You don't have to tell about partners. I don't know if he has others in Colorado. He said he's decided to become straight and marry Susan."

"You mean he's saying his bisexuality is voluntary? He believes he can choose not to ever have sex with men again?"

"That's what he says. I'm not sure. It may really be a choice for him. I'm sure it's not a choice for every homosexual. At least, most of my homosexual patients tell me they never could imagine themselves with women. But anyway, whether he'd stay exclusively with Susan isn't the issue anymore. He should have made that decision before. Now, I think I can tell public health about Susan by name. I think that's legal, but that doesn't guarantee they'll tell her. Anyway, who knows how long it will take to grind through the bureaucracy? The incubation can be as short as six weeks. Maybe she's still okay. His contact was about six weeks ago."

"You couldn't persuade him to tell her?"

"He's really totally irrational about this. He says she's probably got it anyway, so they may as well go down together. I asked him what if she tests negative. He said that didn't matter. I told him that was crazy; she's going to find out sooner or later, maybe by catching it, and then what would that do to a marriage? So he said he'd think about it. That's when I decided to call you. By the time he makes up his mind, it may be too late. Maybe she's still negative. Who knows? Maybe she'll marry him anyway."

"Yeah, maybe she would. But I doubt it. She didn't seem that sure about the relationship. Not so sure as Tim seems to be. She never said fiancé. Maybe she would, but that has to be her choice. I don't think this is going to earn him many Brownie points toward marriage. How am I going to tell her? Got any idea? I'll keep you out of it, but I've got to let her know she's at risk."

"Good. No, I don't know how you're going to do it, but make sure I don't get sued or get in trouble with the board (of medical examiners) for breaking a patient's confidence. Okay?"

"Okay. Thanks."

~

Confidentiality as an ethical obligation dates back to the Hippocratic Oath. There had been much debate in recent years about whether doctors could lawfully break a confidence to warn persons of a threat from a patient whom they were managing medically. The landmark legal case, which began in 1969,[5] involved a student who was under psychiatric care precipitated by rejection by a young woman; the patient told the doctor in August that he was going to kill the girlfriend who had spurned him. The psychiatrist had him held by the campus police, saying that he would sign a temporary hold order because he "was a danger to himself and others." The police found the patient to be rational and stated that he had changed his attitude completely. They released him, and he apparently stopped his psychiatric care at that time. His former girlfriend returned from a trip to Brazil in October, and when he went to her home, she refused to speak with him. He then stabbed her to death, called the police, and awaited their arrival. He was tried and convicted of murder, but an appellate court found fault with jury instructions and changed the conviction to manslaughter. The California Supreme Court found the errors to be so prejudicial that they remanded the case for retrial. Instead, five years after the crime, the state freed him on the condition that he would return to India, his native country, and never return. This he did, and he reportedly was happily married there.

That there is a mate for everyone if they search far enough, however, was not the lesson of the case. The important legal finding came when the girl's parents sued the university and the psychotherapists for the wrongful death of their daughter. This case also struggled through a maze of trials and appeals until the final majority decision—that a physician had a "duty to warn" someone he considered to be in danger. The dissenting judge stressed the idea that breaking the confidence of the mentally ill patient would be a fatal blow to psychotherapy. It would lead to more violence, he stated, because patients with a propensity for violence would not admit it to their doctor and therefore would not be treated in order to reverse that tendency. However, that view was not accepted, and the "duty to warn" has subsequently been extended to contagious diseases, as in AIDS, and genetic diseases. But these extensions, of course, came decades later, when AIDS and genetic information came to the forefront of modern medicine.

At the time of our story, this "duty to warn" was a precedent but was still widely debated because of the dissent. Further confusion arose because this was California common law, and many states, including California, had made special laws directed at AIDS, specifically enforcing confidentiality.

෴

But there I was, wondering how to tell Susan she had to be tested and how to tell her the man she was living with and "getting serious about" had HIV. I had to handle all that, plus protect the internist, who had, with clearly the best of intentions, breached his patient's privacy, then pulled the pin and tossed me this hand grenade. Recall now that it was to be three more years before the FDA (Food and Drug Administration) approved the drug AZT as the first apparently effective drug to treat AIDS. Until then, the general opinion was that AIDS was a death sentence—no questions about "if"; the only question was "when." I called Susan on the phone at the newspaper office. I didn't know what her reaction would be. If I called her at home, Tim would probably be there, and I didn't want to lose a moment in cutting off her contact, at least sexual contact, with him. A colleague called Susan to the phone. She greeted me with, "I've always wanted to say this, so I'm glad you called. What's up doc?"

"Hi, Susan," I responded. "I'm glad you're in a good mood, because I'm going to drop a bomb on you."

"What, I've already got your pap report. It said it was okay. Was that a mistake?"

"No, that's right. It was negative. Susan, can you come to my office?"

"To your office? When? Now?"

"Yes, now. I've got to talk to you seriously, and it's better if we do it face-to-face."

"Wow! What is it? Tell me what it's about. What can be so important that you've got to tell me right now, at the office?"

"Please, come over now and we can talk."

"Okay, okay. I can't even guess, but if you won't tell me on the phone, I'll come over. Should take me half an hour."

"Good. I'll finish up with patients, and we can talk." I was able to see my last appointment and was free to see Susan when she arrived.

"Okay," she said. "What's the mystery?"

"I guess there's no other way to say this, Susan, but you've been exposed to HIV."

"That's impossible." And then in a rush of out-loud thoughts, "I haven't been with anybody else but Tim. You didn't give me any blood, did you? Who? How else? How do you know that? Do *you* have AIDS?"

I reached across the desk and put my hand on her arm. "No," I said. "I don't have AIDS. I just got a call from public health," I lied, "and they told me you were in a list of contacts."

"Who? When?"

"I'm sorry to say, it's Tim."

"Tim? It can't be Tim. We've been living together. We both were tested together. You remember. You sent my blood in."

"There's no mistake, Susan. You'll have to ask Tim, but he may not be willing to talk about it. But there's no mistake," I repeated softly.

She was stunned but held together enough to ask, "So what should I do?"

"Well, we've known each other long enough for me to give you fatherly advice as well as medical. First, let's test you immediately. This is a recent report, and there's a very good chance you may have avoided the disease. It takes a long male-to-female contact to transmit it."

I didn't go into the detail that it is more readily transmitted by anal intercourse because, I quickly concluded to myself, if she had HIV, she had HIV, and by what route didn't matter. "Then," I said, "here comes the fatherly part. I don't know how much you're attached to Tim, but it appears he hasn't been completely honest with you. You need to think the whole thing over, but I would advise you, at the very least, to move out immediately. Certainly, don't have any sexual contact with him until you've had a chance to think long and hard about if he's the man for you."

"Move out? Oh! This is a shocker. How soon do I get my test results? We get along so well. Where did he get it—HIV, I mean?"

"I can't tell you, but it's usually homosexual contact or drug abuse. You aren't into intravenous drugs, are you? Or is Tim? I'm sure you'd be aware of that, wouldn't you? What about those trips to Sausalito?"

She looked pensive. I asked, "Is Tim likely to be violent if you confront him? I mean has he ever hit you or lost it with anyone?"

"No, he's not that kind of person. He's really pretty gentle. I think we can talk. I want to know what's happening. I just don't understand. Was I blind to all this?"

"Well, my best advice is first, move out. Then call him and meet him in a public place to talk about it so you take no chances with his reaction. I've seen the results of too many wives and sweethearts who were assaulted by someone at home. Remember, you thought you knew him well, but you never anticipated this problem. As I said, he hasn't been completely honest with you. I just don't think you should take the chance. You can't predict the reaction of someone who just learned he has a fatal disease and feels he's being rejected. He might be very unstable. And you're not sure, it seems, about your feelings. But you're my patient, so I'm looking out for what I think is best for you. But I'm assuming you wouldn't want to continue this relationship. Is that right?"

"Crap! I don't know. Could he be gay? He's really very nice, but he always was more set on marriage than me. I'm sore because he hasn't been honest. But AIDS! I don't know. I guess I should talk to my folks, although I know what Dad would say. I guess it would be stupid to hitch up with a guy with HIV. But, my God, I may have caught it. I may have AIDS! What was he thinking? What was he thinking?"

⌐

Philosophers who contemplate a certain injustice in the world often advise against precipitous action. Especially, they urge adhering to law and social convention. They recommend instead, "working within the system" to make changes where they seem to be needed. Otherwise, they fear unacceptable social unrest should everyone ignore the rules of society. But periodically, you encounter a situation that calls for anticipation of changes in law and policy that are in the wind but grind too slowly through the legal mill. This was true of the confidentiality laws that were originally written to counter the unjust and often violent reactions by some members of society to victims of AIDS. Merely being identified as having the disease put you at risk of livelihood and often of life. That appears to be an important reason why this disease was treated so differently from other infections by public health authorities. Then it became apparent that uninfected persons were being exposed when it was possible to avoid exposure with prudent forewarning. Some golden mean had to be found between broadcasting the names of HIV patients and keeping a potentially deadly secret. Extant laws were broken, it's true, but in the patient's interest and in anticipation of a wiser resolution.

Three years too late to help me with this dilemma with Susan and Tim, in 1988, the American Medical Association (AMA) finally officially faced the issue of diseases endangering others, particularly in reference to AIDS. The AMA's ethical (not legal) pronouncement was, "We are saying for the first time that, because of the danger to the public health and danger to unknowing partners who may be contaminated with this lethal disease, the physician may be required to violate patient confidentiality. The physician has a responsibility to inform the spouse or known partners. This is more than an option. This is a professional responsibility."

EPILOGUE

Susan had moved out by the time Tim came home. She phoned him that evening, however. When it became apparent to Tim that she was aware of the situation, he tearfully explained the source of the virus and his bisexuality. He also made it clear that he had decided to abstain from homosexual activity and still wanted to marry her. She told him that she was very fond of him, but marriage or any intimate contact was out of the question. Her initial blood tests were negative and negative again at six-month follow-up, demonstrating that the virus had not been transmitted. She had no further sexual contact with him. Later, they met in a coffee shop and had a lengthy talk. Tim, by that time, had accepted reality and had a more rational grip on his situation. She remained part of his support system for several years until he succumbed to pneumonia despite antibiotics and AZT. Not long after, Susan moved to San Diego to work with a newspaper. At her request, I forwarded her medical records to her doctor there.

JENNIE AND LOVE

The first time I saw Jennie, she was upside down and I didn't know her name—I'm an obstetrician and was attending her mother. It was the 1950s, soon after I had started private practice. To me, that was only yesterday, but to a doctor who helps deliver mothers of their babies today, it must seem like the dark ages. No one, including most fathers at that time, even dreamed a father would want to be in the delivery room. There was no imaging by ultrasound, no way to see the baby inside except the relatively crude x-ray. X-rays show bones if they are well-calcified—the mother's better than the baby's—but not much more. Besides, they expose patients to radiation, so we used them as little as possible. Genetic testing was in its infancy, and the denizen of the womb was mostly a mystery until the baby made its debut.

Jennie did not get off to a great start. Her pregnant mom, Doris Blackwell, who lived in Chicago, was visiting her parents in Colorado. She was a little less than a month from her due date when her bag of waters ruptured and she began labor early. She did not have a doctor in Colorado, but her mother was my patient. That's how I came to meet Doris in the delivery room, and very soon thereafter, her brand-new daughter, Jennifer. We had had no foreknowledge of Jennie, so the joyful hubbub that prevailed in the delivery room as Jennie slithered out and I announced, "It's a girl," suddenly turned into conspicuous silence when the nurses and I looked closely at the baby.

"What?" asked Doris, aware of the sudden silence. "What's wrong, Doctor? Is she okay?"

What we had noticed first was the baby's hands, where the fifth finger on each hand was folded into the palm. A quick examination revealed just a single crease that ran completely across each palm (ordinarily, two are present and neither crosses completely from side to side). It's called a simian fold. She had a tiny nose and small ears and seemed a little "floppy" as I placed her in the bassinet. A fold of tissue from the nose to the eyebrow covered a small portion of the white of each eye on the side near the nose—something that would be quite normal in an Asian child. But in this child, these signs suggested that a series of additional abnormalities might be found, which all together are called Down syndrome. In those days, we often called it by an earlier eponym, "Mongolism," suggested by the Asian appearance of the eyes, which had "epicanthal folds."

"There may be a problem, Doris," I equivocated. "Let's let the pediatrician check her out."

Doris strained to lift the upper part of her body and twisted to look at the baby, who was hidden by the warm blanket in the bassinet. "What's wrong? She's not crying much—that's not right, is it? She should be crying. What is it? What's happening?"

"Well," I said, taking a deep breath, "she has some features that look like, uh, what we call Down syndrome." In those days, I blush to confess, it had never occurred to me that her husband might be Asian. As I soon learned, he wasn't.

"Oh," was Doris's barely audible response as she sunk back onto the delivery table, physically and emotionally exhausted. Then, after a pause, "Oh," again as her thoughts expanded into the implications of my words. I looked up to see silent tears streaming down her face as the nurse removed the nasal oxygen from which she had been breathing during the last phases of labor.

"I'm going to have the nurse take her to the nursery and have the pediatrician check her, and then we'll talk. I mean, we'll talk very soon—as soon as he's checked her over and we can tell you all about her, and when your husband is with you. When we're finished here, I'll get him from the waiting room."

That was the beginning—initially a sad beginning—of what turned out ultimately to be an inspiring saga. The excellent pediatrician I had called, on very short notice, took over the task of caring for the baby and explaining Down syndrome to Doris and her husband, Roger. After Doris was discharged from the hospital, I saw her only twice more immediately postpartum, at two weeks, and again at six weeks. Then she and her family (they had another normal child, a boy of three) returned to Chicago, where her husband worked as an attorney for a large corporation. I didn't see Doris or Jennie again for almost twenty years and can take no credit for her wonderful upbringing by remarkable parents. But before I relate how once more I became part of an unusual story, and how together we jumped the gun on the laws about developmental disability and sexuality, I must tell you a little more about Down syndrome.

ↄ

Down syndrome is a genetic condition caused by an extra chromosome number 21. About one in seven hundred to one thousand babies born alive in the United States has this condition. Although these children are developmentally disabled, mental disability varies widely, ranging from severely limited intellect to low average mental capability. The majority function in the mild to moderate range. Jennie had many of the characteristic physical traits of Down syndrome, but none of those features cause disability of themselves. However, these signs herald associated conditions that are variably disabling. Development is slow. Physical abilities, such as walking, and mental abilities, such as using and understanding language, lag behind those of peers without the syndrome. Often, the latter is due to hearing difficulty, that occurs in 60 to 80 percent of Down children. Probably the most serious problem occurs in nearly half the children: malformation of the heart, necessitating risky cardiac surgery. Frequently, intestinal blockage occurs because organs are malformed; such blockages can be fatal unless they are rapidly corrected surgically. Fortunately, the necessary digestive system operations are less hazardous than cardiac surgery. Between 15 and 20 percent of children with Down syndrome have hypothyroidism, which affects overall functioning, particularly of the nervous system.[6] The limpness I noted in Jennie reflected that the ligaments joining many bones are flaccid. Instability of the neck connections is quite common, though it rarely causes serious trouble. Sadly, in those days, few doctors believed these children could lead anything like a normal life; many physicians advised parents to institutionalize the children and get on with their lives as if they hadn't had the child. Happily, Jennie had none of the serious physical abnormalities. And the pediatrician who introduced her to the world did not share the prevailing attitude of pessimism.

But in the 1950s, state or federal aid was minimal to none, unlike today, when laws and regulations provide for special education and "mainstreaming" such children into the regular and special education systems to make their lives as normal as possible. There was no Internet and very few resources that encouraged parents of Down children. So it is greatly to the Blackwells' credit that they were quiet pioneers with Jennie. Her difficulty was mental retardation, a developmental disability that is defined by three factors: IQ score, adaptive functioning, and the age of onset. An IQ test measures and predicts how well individuals learn in their environment. A typical developing child has an IQ between 80 and 119. If the IQ is below 70 to 75, the child must be evaluated regarding mental retardation. Individuals with IQ scores below 75 are subdivided into four levels based on the amount of support they will need: intermittent support (IQ score 55–65), limited support (IQ score 35–55), extensive support (IQ score 25–35), and pervasive support (IQ score 20–25).

Many families dissolve when parents separate as they are faced with caring for a disabled child. Many siblings without handicaps are neglected because so much effort, attention, and resources must be directed to the disabled child. Brothers or sisters remain bitter for a lifetime. Some children are never even conceived, because parents avoid adding another child, even a normal child, to their burden. Other parents find new meaning to their lives and great spiritual fulfillment in their devotion to a developmentally disabled child. Brothers and sisters also may derive a sense of accomplishment from mentoring a less-fortunate sibling. Many families are drawn together in caring for a developmentally disabled child. If only we could match all families with suitable children for their talents, religious attitudes, and resources, both economic and emotional!

Jennie was fortunate to have been born well matched. The Blackwells believed that special tutors, along with their own persistence in stimulating Jennie with readings and regular visits to community activities and museums, would enhance her ability to be a social person. They were right. Today, there is a brighter picture, and support groups that have been formed over the past several decades play a key role.[7]

Unfortunately, these admirable agencies were not in existence when the Blackwells learned how to help Jennie, but that did not deter them.

~

It was not a surprise when Doris and Jennie appeared in my office seventeen years later, because Doris's mother, still my patient, had kept me informed over the intervening years and had arranged the appointment. I could not imagine why they were visiting me and not their Chicago doctor, but I didn't pursue it with Jennie's grandmother. What did surprise me was Jennie. I had attributed to grandmotherly hyperbole the stories related by my patient of Jennie's remarkable progress. It was easy to accept that Jennie was a good-natured and even placid baby. That was conventional wisdom about Down children. But I wondered if that reflected hypothyroidism. I even suggested that, in the next mother-daughter phone call, Doris be asked to have that evaluated.

Intermittently, I had heard of Jennie's desire to do things for herself, starting with simple hygiene, like tooth brushing, and progressing past the complexities of tying shoelaces. I found it difficult to believe the tales of her dancing and, later, even singing. Jennie, I learned, had taken over the task of feeding and walking the friendly family dog from her older brother, who felt these tasks were onerous. They were a joy to Jennie, as she proved she could be relied upon to remember, then carry out recurring responsibilities. She had been interested in helping her mother with household chores and began to show an aptitude for baking—stirring pre-mixed cookies and cakes and listening for the timer to ring and, later, baking from scratch. She was being tutored at home and loved to read, but she did not progress beyond upper-grade-school level. Much of her time was spent listening to the music of Broadway shows, and her grandmother reported she could sing several tunes from *South Pacific* and *Oklahoma*. Later, the Beatles became the focus of her musical attention. This was clearly a girl on the upper scale of retardation whose parents were helping her to realize her very highest potential.

Now, she was almost eighteen years old, and Doris had arranged an appointment for her with me. Both Jennie and Doris had bright smiles as they entered my consulting room. Jennie was small of stature. Someone who was not making a professional appraisal may not have noticed that her gait was just a little broad-based. Her small nose with the flat bridge and the "Asian" eyes were more pronounced than they were at birth. Her ears, and mouth too, had remained relatively small, and her neck was short. But as she came in, she extended her hand, rehearsed some words under her breath and, a moment before Doris introduced us, said aloud, "I am very pleased to meet you, Doctor." Then, after Doris said, "This is Dr. Abrams," she extended her hand again and repeated, "I am very pleased to meet you, Doctor."

"Hi, Jennie. Hello, Doris," I greeted them. "I know you from a long time ago, Jennie," I volunteered. I was pleased to see a comprehending smile cross Jennie's features as she responded, "I know. Mommy told me you were the very first person to see me naked," she giggled.

It certainly sounded like a joke to me, which I did not expect from a person not supposed to be able to think abstractly. "Right," I chuckled. "So," I said, turning back and forth between Doris and Jennie, "what brings you to see me after all these years?"

"Well," said Doris, looking down at her hands, now folded in her lap, "it's pretty complicated, but I'll try to explain it all." Then, looking up directly at me, she said, "I hope you've put lots of time aside. It's a long story."

"Sure," I replied. "We've got lots of catching up to do."

"Let me start sort of at the end. Jennie has a really nice boyfriend. She met him two years ago at the Special Olympics. He is two years older than Jennie, and he lives near us in Chicago. He has a paying job at a gym keeping the locker room in order and handing out towels and some of the equipment. Roger and I have taken them out together to musical events, plays, movies, and things. They've also been alone in Jennie's room, listening to records and TV." Then she turned, put her hand on Jennie's arm, and looked back at me, evidently feeling she had to ward off criticism. "But then, someone else has always been home with them."

I had watched Jennie nodding and smiling appropriately as her mother related the history and began to have a dreadful feeling about where this was headed. I hoped they weren't going to tell me that Jennie was pregnant and had come to Colorado for an abortion. Colorado had been the first state to legalize abortion, in 1967. At the time we were consulting, it was not yet legal in Illinois.

Doris continued, "It had been several years before this when Jennie had become aware that she was different from many of the children she watched on television. I think it started when reading became so hard for her. We explained, and I think she understood, that some things were too hard for her to do but that there were other areas where she could really shine. The Special Olympics were great for her, and she had won several events."

Jennie enthusiastically offered, "I could play because I have Down syndrome and I got medals and hugs from Coach Arbeit and Ms. Gordon. But tell him more about George, Mommy, George and me."

"Okay, Jennie." Doris went on, "At first, Jennie was confused when this happened because we had spoken to her previously about good and bad touching and affection, and coaches aren't family. Right, Jennie?" Turning back to me, she continued, "Then she told me that she especially liked it when George—that's her boyfriend—hugged her when she won a medal. Then he hugged her when she hadn't won a medal."

Looking back, I'm embarrassed that I broke my own rule about not interrupting a patient when she is relating a history. Nevertheless, at that point I couldn't keep my professional cool because I had to find out if Jennie was pregnant, and I interjected, "Do you know about babies, Jennie?"

Doris answered, "We talked about that when menstruation began, baby making and all that, and we explained what kind of touching and affection was okay and what situations to avoid. You know what's okay, don't you, Jennie?"

"Yes, but I want to hug George. I like to hug George. It feels very nice. We want to make love naked, like in the book Jimmie has under his mattress. George said so too," Jennie announced matter-of-factly.

I couldn't hold back, "But did you do that, Jennie? Are you going to have a baby?"

Jennie and Doris spoke simultaneously. Jennie shook her head vigorously, saying, "I don't want to," and Doris quickly replied, "Oh, no."

"Then what—?"

Doris continued, "We all agree Jennie shouldn't have a baby, because she knows she can't take proper care of a baby. Right, Jennie?"

Jennie nodded, and I asked, "Is that right, Jennie? Don't you think you can take care of a baby? You seem pretty responsible to me."

Doris looked at me as if I were an incarnation of malevolence or, at the very least, insane. But I wanted to know how much of this venture truly indicated Jennie's feeling rather than just parroted answers without true understanding. I pressed on. "Is that the way you truly feel, Jennie? You don't want a baby? Don't you think you could take care of a baby?"

"I can't and I won't. Positively and absolutely and totally beyond the shadow of a doubt," was Jennie's astonishing reply.

Wow! I thought. Too literate and stereotyped, but regardless of where she had heard the phrases before, certainly emphatic and very convincing. Still wondering where that litany had come from, I asked, "So where do I come in? How can I be of help?"

Doris forged on resolutely, "We would like you to do a tubal ligation."

"But why here?" I asked, secretly relieved that was what they were seeking rather than what I had speculated previously. "Why did you have to come to Colorado? Why didn't you ask your doctor back home?"

"Two reasons," said Doris. "First, my Chicago doctor won't do any sterilizations for anyone because of his religion."

"He's Catholic," Jennie chimed in.

Doris grimaced slightly and went on. "Second, when Jennie was born, you and the Denver pediatrician were really understanding and forward-looking about Down children." She paused and finished in a rush, "I thought you'd be more likely to believe they ought to be able to have as full a life as possible, and that, when they were old enough, that certainly should include love and affection and sex. There!" She exhaled sharply and sagged in her chair as if relieved of a physical burden.

⌐

That was a novel idea, rarely expressed at that time. Sterilization for the developmentally disabled in the United States has gone through three phases. A eugenic enthusiasm for sterilization, not only of the developmentally disabled but also thousands of others deemed socially unfit, was the shameful phase one. The second phase was a backlash against sterilization, opposing it either on religious grounds or for fear of violating civil liberties, regardless of how appropriate and carefully selected. The third and most recent phase is recognition that in special circumstances, it adds immensely to the quality of life for those who wish to be intimate but are sufficiently aware that rearing children will always be beyond their capability. Therefore, they choose or at least assent to being sterilized.

The first phase remains an embarrassment in the history of our most respected institutions, a time when law and medicine went far astray. The American eugenics movement demonstrated the synergy that can develop when an ounce of science is mixed with a ton of zealotry. In the early part of the twentieth century, the movement developed, supported by a heterogeneous group of doctors, scientists, judges, wealthy American businessmen, politicians, anti-immigration legislators, law enforcement personnel, racists, and misled philanthropists.[8] Beginning with Indiana in 1907, thirty state legislatures were persuaded to pass laws permitting "involuntary asexualization."[9] They did not distinguish between sterilization and castration. Ill-informed, self-proclaimed, and badly mistaken experts convinced legislators that there were inherited conditions they called congenital pauperism, congenital prostitution, congenital degeneracy, and congenital criminality—preposterous and unscientific assertions. Epilepsy, feeblemindedness, and insanity were grouped together as indications for sterilization, supposedly to avoid future generations with these afflictions.

One of the most prominent spokesmen was a Dr. Davenport, who preached that society could eliminate costly burdens through a program of mandatory sterilization. He wrote in 1911, "It is a reproach to our intelligence that we as a people, proud in other aspects of our control of nature, should have to support about half a million insane, feebleminded, epileptic, blind and deaf, eighty thousand prisoners and one hundred thousand paupers at a cost of over one hundred million dollars per year."[10]

As state after state succumbed to this rhetoric, Supreme Court Justice Oliver Wendell Holmes added legitimacy to it with the infamous Buck v. Bell decision in 1929. Carrie Buck, the eighteen-year-old illegitimate daughter of an allegedly feebleminded mother, herself gave birth to a child. Carrie reportedly had the mental age of nine. This assessment was disproved by interviews with her later, when she was a mature woman. Her daughter, at age seven months, was reported to be feebleminded by a social worker. Later, the child was found to develop quite normally in school until she died at age eight from an intestinal infection.

Schoolteacher and self-anointed expert Harry Laughlin was a prolific author and speaker on the subject of eugenics. He was asked to review Carrie's records. Without seeing the patient, he stated that she was a member of the "shiftless, ignorant, and worthless class of antisocial whites" and that the possibility of her feeblemindedness being due to nonhereditary causes was "exceptionally remote." Carrie's lawyer, in his prophetic brief, noted the peril to society if the sterilization law was upheld, warning, "A reign of doctors will be inaugurated and in the name of science new classes will be added, even races may be brought within the scope of such a regulation and the worst forms of tyranny may be practiced."[11]

In the appeal to the Supreme Court, the law was upheld in the oft-quoted phrase of Justice Holmes, "three generations of imbeciles are enough."[12] Subsequent follow-up has demonstrated that at least one and possibly two of these three generations were quite normal.

In the United States, the beginning of the backlash that followed, which made all sterilization taboo, was in reaction to the excesses of Nazi Germany. Sterilization laws were passed in Germany in 1933 (twenty-six years after Indiana's law) following careful study of California's law. It would be unfair not to mention that other European countries, such as Sweden, Finland, Norway, and Denmark, also passed sterilization eugenics laws. That Scandinavian countries were involved with eugenics first appeared to reach public attention in 1997. However, Germany carried its program far beyond sterilization. The government and the medical profession together murdered thousands of its own citizens for "severe mental defect or illness," including epilepsy and other conditions having only the remotest possible connection with genetics. So many retarded children died of "pneumonia" after transfer from home to public or private medical institutions that the program of eugenic murder (sometimes misnamed "euthanasia"), begun in 1940, was terminated in 1942 due to internal public outcry from the German citizens themselves. The foremost scientist who led Germany's program in this field, Fritz Lenz, chided his German colleagues in 1923 for being far behind America in matters of racial purity and eugenics.[13]

Despite a U.S. Supreme Court ruling in 1942[14] establishing a fundamental right to procreation, and in spite of substantial opposition to the eugenics movement in the United States right from the beginning, sterilization continued on eugenic grounds until 1972.

The backlash was strongly evidenced in 1974 by a legal case involving involuntary sterilization of two black children under sixteen years of age. This case resulted in a moratorium on federal financing of sterilization of anyone under twenty-one years of age.[15] Concerns about racism and legal age of consent were both important factors reinforcing the movement against sterilization, regardless of the presence of valid medical indications.

It was not until 1981 that a legal process for sterilization of mentally retarded minors was established in Colorado; Doris and Jennie and I were trying to deal with this dilemma several years before this guideline was settled.[16] It never occurred to me to consult a lawyer. Doctors then were more inclined to make difficult decisions based on medical reasoning rather than legal considerations. We were not involved with any government financing. Hospital ethics committees would be established many years into the future, with most being founded in the 1980s and beyond. So we proceeded as common sense dictated and anticipated the process that was later approved by society.

First, I wrestled with the idea of alternative contraception. Intrauterine devices (IUDs) usually increased menstrual flow, often caused cramping, sometimes led to serious infection, and were difficult to place in the uterus of a patient who had never been pregnant. Pills were available but were not without side effects, especially considering the unknowns of a lifetime of taking hormones. Jennie could probably be relied upon to take them properly, but that was unpredictable, especially if she became nauseated. A relatively simple surgical procedure, laparoscopic tubal occlusion, had no aftereffects, and Jennie could go home a few hours following the procedure. This was a surgical procedure for which consent was necessary; it was considered to be permanent but was sometimes reversible with more surgery.

It was apparent that we could not get a true informed consent from a minor, especially one who was admittedly mentally retarded. I sought a written consultation from a psychiatrist who worked with the developmentally disabled, and from our pediatrician to evaluate Jennie's capability to understand what we were proposing. I asked a special education teacher with a degree in social work who worked exclusively with the mentally retarded to interview her and comment on the whole idea while evaluating Jennie's grasp of the proposal. There was no doubt that we had Jennie's assent and cooperation. The two people who cared most about her, her mother and father, appeared to genuinely have her best interest at heart. Their judgment was very important because they had brought her along to a remarkable stage, far beyond what might have been predicted at her birth. They were remarkably enlightened regarding her capacity and need for love and affection, which she now wanted to express in a more adult way.

All the consultants concurred that Jennie functioned at the upper level of the retardation scale. They indicated that she was capable, at her level of understanding, of consenting—in fact, desiring—what was being proposed; she knew that the procedure would enable her to express the love a mature postpubertal child feels toward another. They also agreed that, advanced as she was in some aspects of daily living, bearing and raising a child was beyond her capabilities and that there was no expectation that her mental aptitude would change.

It took several days to complete the evaluation simply because Jennie had to travel around town to the different consultants. When she returned for what I hoped would be a preoperative session with me, I asked her what she thought about so many people questioning her. I told her I wanted to be sure she was completely aware of what we all had planned together, so I also asked if she would explain to me what it was all about.

"They were nice," she said. "Their job is—they all work with people like me who are a little slow. It's special to talk with people who know that I don't have all the words to tell them, to tell them about how I feel, but they know anyway. They all asked lots of the same questions, though. I should have spoken with them all at once.

But the best thing was they said I could make love, but I didn't have to have a baby if I didn't want one, and I told them I don't want one. I like babies, but sometimes I don't do everything right, and you can't take chances with a real baby. I don't have to have a baby if I don't want to."

I suppose I shouldn't be surprised, as I almost always am, by flashes of insight evidenced by mentally retarded persons. Their thought processes are so literal and direct that it's invariably when you least expect it somewhat abstract concepts are voiced. Jennie may not have been competent in a legal sense, but she seemed to know very well what we had been evaluating and the consequences of the planned intervention.

None of the consultants had questioned the propriety of this seventeen-year-old having sexual relations. Certainly, a seventeen-year-old is physiologically ready. Sexual relations at any age are not *intrinsically* immoral. It varies with the culture. The objection in our culture is the adolescent's inability to deal with consequences such as pregnancy, a devastating breakup with a severe impact on feelings of self-worth, the risk of sexually transmitted disease, their peer pressures, or the potential for abuse or exploitation. With the concern for pregnancy removed—and Jennie's and George's single-minded attachment to each other—the hazards that make it taboo for some segments of our society did not seem as pertinent.

After explaining to Jennie, Doris, and Jennie's father, Roger, exactly the procedure for anesthesia and surgery, including warnings about needle sticks and postoperative pains, they all signed consent forms, even though Jennie couldn't, technically. But I wanted to make her aware of how important it was that she understand this was an occasion of consequence. I believed that, by putting her signature on an official document, she would appreciate that everyone thought this was truly special.

❦

I thought I had dotted all the *i*'s and crossed all the *t*'s when I arrived in the operating area the morning of surgery, but I had not counted on Ms. Martin. Operating rooms are replete with regulations designed to eliminate human error from this area of critical interventions. To be as certain of this as possible, a dictator is anointed and called the head operating room nurse. Ms. Martin was one such individual. In the interest of efficiency and safety, the surgeons, with bent knee, bowed head and pledges of eternal fealty—submit. As I came through the door, there was Ms. Martin scowling at me and waving a paper.

Skipping the formality of a greeting, she announced, "You can't sterilize a seventeen-year-old girl."

My reply was delivered gently. "Have you read the rest of the chart, or did you just go straight to the consent form?"

"It doesn't matter," she retorted. "You can't sterilize a seventeen-year-old."

"Please, Ms. Martin, let's read the chart together, then let's go to the holding area and meet Jennie and her parents."

We retrieved the chart, and I pointed out the consultations from three reputable specialists, each of whom had particular expertise with the developmentally disabled. I watched her as she read the unique story of Jennie's birth and maturation—as far as maturation could go. Her brow furrowed as she read one after the other, and then she looked up and asked, "Is this legal?"

"Well," I replied, "it isn't illegal. And it makes a lot of sense."

"Doesn't she have to be twenty-one?"

"It wouldn't make it any more legal, and that gives her three more unprotected years to get pregnant. She's never going to be capable of having and rearing a baby—everyone agrees, and she does too. So why block real attachment and affection between two disadvantaged people. We're trying to make sure they both get as much out of life as possible." I could see her wavering, so I added, "I'll take full responsibility and even write down that you are opposed."

"Well, now that I've read the story, I'm not really opposed, but write it down anyway so when the legal eagles get on my tail, I have something to point to."

"You have a heart of gold, Ms. Martin."

EPILOGUE

Several years later, a Colorado court decision established a procedure, not unlike the process that we had improvised, for sterilization of the developmentally disabled, with provisions for those who are competent as well as for minors.[17] The ethics committee of The American College of Obstetricians and Gynecologists (ACOG) also created a policy addressing this circumstance, endorsing sterilization when it is appropriate for carefully evaluated patients who they described as the "retarded." They qualified their terminology, indicating no disrespect was meant by using the term "retarded," but that was the terminology widely understood at the time.[18] In 1999, the American Academy of Pediatrics (AAP) updated their previous statement, also entitled "Sterilization of Women Who Are Mentally Handicapped," concurring in the essential elements of the ACOG policy.[19]

CELESTE

I must confess I didn't like Betty's choice when she came to me with her decision. Nevertheless, I never had any question in my mind that it was her decision to make. I had tried to hide my bias. I had told her that whatever she decided, I would support her fully and without reservation. That blithe resolution was tested sorely as her pregnancy progressed, at least the "without reservation" part.

I had better explain why we had different views, so I'll start with the day Betty Wroshaw came in for her first prenatal visit. Betty had married later than usual, and she had her first child when she was thirty-three. She and her husband had become anxious after the birth of their first child because they had been trying for four years to get a little sister or a little brother for their daughter, Amy. Betty had missed her second menstrual period when she came in. She was excited but concerned because it had taken so long.

In 1995, we often did a quick ultrasound scan, often on the first visit, to be sure about the reason for the skipped periods. We could show that there was a pregnancy and make sure that it was alive because we were able to demonstrate a heartbeat. Unfortunately, today a good deal of medical practice is guided by what insurance pays for, and they usually pay for only one ultrasound scan. Most obstetricians had their own scanner in their office, so we didn't charge for that first scan, because we knew there would be another more extensive one later. But if the patient had to be sent outside to an imaging center, there would be a charge, so some patients just had to wait and see, or pay for an "extra" scan. A full-term pregnancy is usually calculated as forty weeks from the first missed menstrual period. Today, the practice most often is to postpone a routine scan until halfway—twenty weeks. If you're going to do only one, you get the most information for the money at that stage of pregnancy.

Not many men accompany their wife to an obstetrician's office. They feel out of place there. The mere fact that Betty's husband had come with her to my office, knowing that he would be surrounded by pregnant women in the waiting room, showed how deeply he was invested in the pregnancy. I was pleased to tell them both that they were off to a good start. We did initial basic blood and urine tests. Betty was already on a prenatal vitamin, which she had continued since her first pregnancy, including proper amounts of folic acid to prevent nervous system abnormalities. We set up her next visit for four weeks later, about eleven weeks of pregnancy.

Her next visit was uneventful, with good blood pressures, little weight gain, and a report that she had had virtually no nausea, a symptom that had plagued her first pregnancy. She also mentioned something that only in retrospect did I realize might have been a little forewarning of problems to come. She jokingly said she was a little "pouchy"—that she hadn't expected to be showing so early, especially compared to her first pregnancy, when no one could tell until at least six months, "maybe even seven."

At about fifteen weeks of pregnancy, we drew a triple-screen blood test from Betty's arm.[20] The results of the blood test gave us the first real indication that all was not well. The test is for three different hormones and protein markers in the mother's serum. Their levels in combination can indicate the status of the fetus,[21] and the results are used to predict occult abnormalities, such as defects in the formation of the brain and spinal cord, as well as twinning or chromosomal errors associated with genetic anomalies. The pattern that we found was suggestive of a serious abnormality in chromosome number 18. Chromosomes normally come in pairs, but the pattern of three low levels suggested this chromosome was tripled—there was an extra chromosome—and that finding foretold the probability of many malformations in Betty's baby-to-be. I called her on the phone that evening and told her that her blood test showed there might be something wrong.

"What? What do you mean, something wrong?"

"I can't be sure yet, Betty," I replied, "but if your dates are right, there may be some problems with the baby."

"Like what? What could be wrong?"

"I promise I'll go into all the details after we do one more test, an ultrasound, and that can show us what may be wrong, if anything is at all."

"Can't you give me some idea? I mean how serious could it be?"

"Well, again, could your dates be off? Are you sure when you became pregnant? Because the tests mean different things, depending on how far along you are."

"No, my dates are right. Ted and I have been keeping track for so long now that making love has become a little mechanical. But the dates are accurate and my periods are regular. So what could be wrong?"

"Well, I don't want to jump to any conclusions—we really should talk after the ultrasound—but it could be tripling of a chromosome, and that might indicate something quite serious, like a malformed heart that doesn't function properly or some other organs that can't do their vital jobs."

"Oh!" She paused for a moment to digest the significance of the lab findings and my conjecture about the possibilities they raised. "Okay, when can I get the ultrasound?" Then, with determination, she went on, "And Doctor, we haven't talked about this yet, and it's very important that we understand each other. I believe God has a plan for everybody, and I've always trusted that wherever God leads me is right. I want to be very clear about this—no matter what you find, I will do everything I can to have this baby."

"Of course, Betty. But we're getting way ahead of ourselves. Let's see what the ultrasound shows. Come in tomorrow, after three."

That statement about God's plan helped me understand why Betty had not sought medical help as the years passed without her achieving the much-desired pregnancy. I guessed she had simply trusted that if God's plan included a pregnancy, she would become pregnant without outside intervention—and indeed she had. I didn't want to agitate Betty any further, so I refrained from telling her what I believe: I'm not at all sure there is a plan, but if there is, I believe doctors, and whatever they have to offer, are part of it. Of course, both of these ideas are "beliefs." There's no way of proving either of them.

The three of us met first in my consulting room the next day. Ted had come along for the ultrasound. I explained that we would go into a darkened room with a female technician who would guide the handheld probe. The probe, I told them, resembled in shape a small flashlight and was lubricated with a warm gel that let it glide gently over the exposed abdomen. Inaudible sound waves were translated via the probe into a live picture on a screen much like a computer monitor or TV screen. I asked them if they wanted an explanation as we saw things on the screen in "real time"; or, if they preferred, they could wait for a more complete analysis, after I studied the pictures that we would take as we progressed through the scan. I told them I wasn't sure what we would see, but that we were looking for certain body formations typical of the chromosome abnormality I suspected, trisomy 18. They chose to hear information as it was revealed.

Awesome is a word tossed about much too casually by the young people we know. It should be reserved for such amazing advances as the ability to look inside the pregnant uterus. Thousands of years have gone by with myriads of modes of speculative augury predicting the characteristics of the inhabitant of the uterus. Gender was foretold by the direction a wedding ring swung on a string suspended over the belly, or by whether the abdomen protruded "high" or "low," "in front" or "behind." Birthmarks were forecast if strawberries or grapes were part of the mother's diet. Malformations were deemed almost inevitable if the mother viewed certain animals in proximity to delivery or if a sudden fright had occurred. In some cultures, knives were taboo for pregnant women. But with ultrasound, the abdominal wall and the womb had become virtually transparent, allowing accurate visualization of the physical characteristics of the baby before it made its entry into the world of lungs and breath.

I started my description. "I see more fluid than I would expect at this stage. That's probably why you felt you were showing pretty early. You're really sure about the dates, aren't you?"

"Yes," she answered in a subdued voice that reflected her emotional state.

"And I can tell you for sure that you have a little girl." I thought to myself, *That's another strike—nearly 80 percent of trisomy 18 babies are girls.* "She is a little small for the dates. The foot has a shape we call "rocker bottom." See, from the side, it's like the arc on the bottom of a rocking chair."

As the probe moved smoothly across the abdominal contours, a hand came into view. The fist was clenched, and the fifth and fourth fingers folded across the neighboring fingers. That was very characteristic of the chromosome number 18 defect. I thought, *Maybe this ongoing narration is too much at once. A short breather might be better,* so I said, "I'm not sure this is the best way to talk to you about your baby—I mean, lying on your back in a dark room. Should I go on?"

"It's really better this way. Then you can't see me cry." Her tremulous voice witnessed what our eyes couldn't see in the dim light cast from the shadowy screen.

I went on. "Well, the hand—see here, the last two fingers are folded toward the middle, over the fingers next to them? That's a very strong marker for trisomy 18."

Ted asked, "Can't that be fixed? I mean with surgery or something?"

"It's not that, Ted, not the hands. They are just the marker, the telltale sign of everything else that goes along with trisomy 18. That's the really bad part."

"What do you mean?" he asked.

"I just don't know any easy way to tell you this, but if we confirm this with chromosome testing, then the survival statistics are very bleak. Let's see if we can see the baby's heart now." We moved the probe until we could see the heart. It was difficult because it was very early in the pregnancy, but the heart did not look normal. We couldn't see the four chambers, which, in turn, receive blood with low oxygen, pump it through the lungs to become oxygenated, and then recirculate it through the body. "Well, I'm not absolutely sure now," I said, "but if it is what I'm almost certain it is, then we will find a heart problem. More than 90 percent of trisomy 18 babies have heart abnormalities. We can recheck it later if you decide to continue the pregnancy."

"I did tell you that there's no question about that, Doctor," Betty replied firmly. "We have no intention at all of resisting God's wishes for us and for our baby. We know we are not wise enough to understand all of God's plan, but we simply put our trust in Him as we always have, and we know this will be a blessing, whatever happens."

"Then, even though you wouldn't terminate the pregnancy, if we suspect that diagnosis, I think it would be useful to do an amniocentesis," I suggested, "because it will help you prepare for the likely outcome with the baby. After you get dressed, we can arrange the amnio—if you want one." I left the ultrasound room and set up an amniocentesis for the next day, knowing I could cancel if she decided against it.

When the couple returned to the consultation room, I told them I'd like to explain more about trisomy 18. "Are you ready to hear more about the baby's diagnosis today, Betty, or have you had enough for one day? I know this has been a shock, even though we've been coming upon it bit by bit."

"For now, Doctor, I just want to know one main thing. Will my baby live?"

"I'm sorry I can't give you a better answer and be more precise, but I can only cite statistics. Later, another ultrasound when the baby is bigger can make us a little more accurate, but every baby is different. Unfortunately, many of these babies don't survive to birth, even if no one interferes. But anyway, statistically, only half survive beyond a week after birth and 90 percent are gone by six months. Only 10 percent survive the first year. To be honest, many mothers opt for abortion. There may be many different reasons, but some feel with such poor odds, they'd sooner start a new pregnancy rather than going through a whole pregnancy with such a dismal prognosis. I must tell you also that it's not necessarily an absolutely lethal condition, although the death rate is very high. There are a very few babies who have lived to childhood and rarely, even to adulthood. Much will depend on what defect we find in the heart, because heart failure is a main cause of death. There also can be something wrong with the brain signals to the lungs, because some of these babies just seem to forget to breathe."

Ted spoke up for the first time. "I guess we're both overwhelmed with this news, Doctor, but what I'm concerned with mostly—is there any risk to Betty?"

"No more than any other pregnancy, Ted," I replied.

"Because I don't see things exactly the way Betty does," he continued.

"What do you mean?" I asked.

"Well, I guess you could say Betty is a lot more religious than I am. I don't usually go to church with her. Not that I don't believe in God, because I do, but I also believe God doesn't mean for us to just lie back and put everything in Jesus' hands. I mean he gave us brains to think with so we can do things that we think are right. We can change things if we need to—not just accept things that come our way—if we can do something to make them better. Know what I mean?"

"Sure I do, Ted, but—I know you've heard of Watson and Crick?"

"Sure, the DNA helix—they were the ones who figured it out, right?"

"Right, and I would guess they've thought long and hard about what their discovery led to—genetic engineering and manipulations with chromosomes, that sort of thing. Well, Watson was asked about who should be in charge of decisions now that we have learned so much more about chromosomes." I asked rhetorically, "You know what he said? He said, 'I think all genetic decisions should be made by women—not the state, not their husbands, just by women—

because they're going to give birth to those children, and they're going to be the ones most responsible.' I agree with him. Oh sure, we husbands and fathers have input; in fact, we should have lots of input. But in the last analysis, we have to remember the geography. You can't really separate mother and baby. At least not at this stage. The hard work is theirs, and I believe they should have the last word, too. In the end, I always go with the mother's decision."

Betty said quietly, "Ted, you know how important this is to me. I've already prayed and put myself in His hands, and I'm going to trust that Jesus will watch over me and our baby and even you, whether you go to church or not. Let's talk things over at home and come in for the amnio, and then we'll know enough to make plans insofar as God wills. I will pray, and he will guide me to do what is right. And remember, we are not certain that there are really serious problems yet."

We left it at that. I didn't say any more about how very serious this was, because it is better to let people build up their defenses gradually against a terrible situation, even if there is an element of denial that eases things temporarily. I was grateful that Betty had such strong faith. Most doctors will testify that things are handled much better by patients with deep-seated beliefs. She was going to be tested soon.

The next day, after explaining the risks (about one in a two hundred to four hundred chance for miscarriage) and obtaining consent, I proceeded with the amniocentesis. Using local anesthesia and guided by ultrasound visualization of the amniotic sac, I inserted a long, slender needle and withdrew a few teaspoons of slightly yellow-tinged fluid. This fluid was sent to the lab for chromosome analysis; the analysis would ascertain whether the baby's cells found in the fluid showed three chromosomes instead of two in the number 18 position. In less than two weeks, we had the answer. The chromosome analysis did show the abnormal trisomy, and that put us on the track we followed past the birth of baby Celeste Wroshaw.

Again, Betty, Ted, and I met. Betty asked, "Is it what you thought it was?"

"Yes, trisomy 18."

Betty started to speak, saying, "We looked it up, Ted and I, and—" but she couldn't hold back the tears. "Sorry, I thought we had gone over it enough so I wouldn't cry now, talking to you about it, but—" Betty stopped speaking as she began to weep. Ted put his arm around her, and his face showed the distress he felt as his wife sobbed. I always had tissues on my desk and I slid the box over to her. She plucked several from the container, wiped her tears, blew her nose, and said, "There, I'm done." I waited. She looked up at me and said, "I read that so many things can go wrong, it's no wonder so many babies die. They can have an abnormal heart, blocked bowels, poorly functioning or absent kidneys—you can't live without kidneys, can you?"

"No, you can't. But we already know your baby has kidneys. We don't know if they're going to work. If the baby survives to be born, she has a 40 percent chance of living for a month. From that group, about one in twenty might live for a year. Of those few survivors, one in a hundred might survive to ten. And out of that small number comes the rare ones who survive into their twenties or beyond."

"So what can we do to make her one of those survivors?" Ted exhorted, still seeking a way to fly in the face of misfortune, unwilling yet to accept that no medical miracle was forthcoming.

"Nothing now, but depending on what we find on the next ultrasound, we may be able to predict what's most likely. But if she has several lethal abnormalities, then only being able to fix some would put her through unnecessary pain, unless we could fix them all."

When Betty next came in for a prenatal visit—this time without Ted, who was at work—she told me of the difficulties she was experiencing, knowing her baby would probably not survive. Soon she would begin to show she was pregnant, and friends would be joyous about the "blessed event." She knew how painful it would be for everyone when she explained—and she didn't want to explain over and over again. She hadn't told Amy, her four-year-old, about the pregnancy, and she was trying to think about what she should be told and when. It was not likely that Amy would even notice her mother was pregnant unless it was called to her attention. I suggested that she should wait a little longer, that many decisions could be made better after the ultrasound. I was especially interested in what we could see about the heart, I explained, because some abnormalities are absolutely incompatible with life outside the womb. Inside the womb, the placenta acts like a heart-lung machine, bringing the oxygen necessary for life. If the baby's heart couldn't do that, once she was outside the womb, she could live only minutes or hours.

"I'm not trying to push you or anything, Betty, but I'm going to ask you again because timing can be important. If you knew your baby couldn't survive more than a few hours after delivery, would you terminate the pregnancy? Don't be angry with me; the reason I'm asking again is because the earlier a pregnancy is terminated, the safer it is for you. I'd do the ultrasound sooner if termination were still an option."

"I'm afraid you really don't understand, Doctor," Betty replied, with a touch of reproach and exasperation in her voice. "You are used to approaching difficulties from a technical viewpoint. You're speaking about what looks like the best medical solution to a medical problem, and I'm glad that you know so much about being a good doctor. But you know? This isn't a medical problem to me. This is my baby and I love her already. You mustn't value a life by measuring its length. What you said to Ted the other day was very important to me. You said that in the end, these choices are up to the mother. I hope you meant that."

"Of course I meant that, Betty, but I really have to tell you what we can do medically and what is my best medical advice. You know there are so many different ways to approach quandaries and more than one may be okay. We may have different values and beliefs—I think we do—but that won't prevent me from helping you in the way you want to be helped, unless it's a real violation of my ethics. So if it's okay with you, I'll go on telling you what I think, but I will respect your decisions. I wouldn't have a clear conscience if I thought you were doing the wrong thing and I didn't say anything."

"I think that's fair, Doctor. You present my options and I'll choose. But don't leave anything out, even if it's not your first choice."

At about twenty weeks, we did a definitive ultrasound. It showed a malformed heart with abnormal valves that couldn't function as they should to keep the blood circulating adequately. There was also a hole between the chambers that deflected the normal pattern of flow. Ted was with us this time as I told them about the heart. "I'm afraid the heart is not going to be able to sustain the baby once she is born," I said. "I can't tell you if the kidneys will work or if there's anything wrong with the brain. That won't show on any test. We just have to wait and see. But I must be honest; if she lives long enough to be born—and she may not—I think she'll only survive minutes or hours."

They came from the imaging room to my office, and Ted said, "Betty's been a mess, Doctor. Can you give her something?"

Betty's voice was husky but firm. She said, "Ted, I told you I wasn't going to take any medicines while I was pregnant. I'll be okay. I was ready for today, although I hoped it would be different. I'm just going to pray a little harder, and I've decided to send a card to our good friends at church and on our block explaining what's happened and that I intend to go as far as God lets me with the baby. I believe God put this precious baby into our hands for a reason. Other parents might not care for her the way we will. We will love her and hold her and do whatever we can to help her live whatever life God intended. And if she dies, we will have done what was right for her until she becomes the angel I know God intends her to be."

Ted's lips tightened and his brow furrowed. He turned to me and asked, "What do you think, Doctor? Do you think she should continue on with the pregnancy?"

Betty looked startled by Ted's question. She said a little angrily, "I thought we had settled that, Ted."

I quickly replied, "Ted, it's not important what I think. What do you think?"

To the astonishment of both Betty and me, Ted put his face in his hands and began to sob. When she saw that, Betty dissolved into tears. And confronted with this scene, I discovered copious tears running down my own cheeks. I found myself standing alongside of Ted in his chair with a hand across his bowed shoulders, dabbing my face and handing out tissues to my patients. We looked at each other, and all of us began a gurgling mixture of laughter and tears and then handclasps and hugs all around. Sometimes, I found, losing professional aplomb has a place.

"Ted, you've been hanging tough through all of this," I said, "and obviously it's hit you hard and you've had no outlet. It's important that everyone shares their feelings in a difficult situation like this, and we'll all try to support each other. It looks as if Betty's faith is good for her, and you can feel free to come talk to me, if you can brave a waiting room full of women."

We shed a good deal of tension that day and gained a renewed confidence in pursuing the course that *I* thought was set by Betty and that *Betty* thought was set by God. The months crept by, and the baby continued to move sufficiently to reassure Betty. About a month from term, we again sat in my office.

"What have you told Amy?" I asked.

"I explained that her new baby sister—who, by the way, we've named Celeste—might become an angel before or just after she's born. Either way, she'll be in heaven with Jesus and we'll all meet there someday, and Celeste will be whole and healthy then."

"How did she deal with that?"

"No problem. It's what she's heard before about Grandma Wroshaw. In fact, she was pleased that the baby would be with Grandma and they were both starting to live forever with Jesus."

"Good. I'm sure your mind is more at ease. You were worried about how she'd take the disappointment." I went on, "Today, I want to talk about delivery. More than half of these babies are delivered by caesarian section, but that's because they're not always diagnosed in advance and when there are signs of fetal distress—which occur very frequently—they're delivered surgically. I don't think we should do that."

↩

I found myself in the unusual situation of asking a patient for permission *not* to operate.

Doctors one hundred or even fifty years ago would not have found themselves in this position. They would have simply done what they thought was best in their judgment, and no one would have questioned them. A patient who sought a doctor's help would have known that she had put the doctor in complete and unchallenged control of the situation. Informed consent was a revolutionary change in the doctor-patient relationship. It's so much a part of Western medical practice today that we don't think of it as an innovation, much less the legal and ethical standard it has become. The idea of patient participation in decisions is very recent. Looking backward, one can't find a principle that grew from antiquity into today's doctrine of informed consent. In fact, you'll find just the opposite. For centuries, the "doctor knows best" principle of paternalism prevailed.

Hippocrates[22] advised "concealing most things from the patient...revealing nothing of the patient's future or present condition." Cicero advised everyone not to warn others of impending danger if there was nothing that could be done to avoid it. The French medieval surgeon Henri de Mondeville advised his colleagues to "Promise a cure to every patient, but tell [only] the parents or friends if there is any danger." He also recommended exaggerating the problem or minimizing it—whichever was necessary to get the patient to comply with the doctor's orders.

Thomas Percival published a definitive work on medical ethics in England a year before his death in 1804. He chose always to lie to a patient with a terminal illness, and any other time he felt the truth would cause harm. He considered lying not a lack of fidelity to the patient but rather a sacrifice the doctor had to make, regrettably forced upon him by his role that demanded deception in the name of "professional justice and social duty."

The AMA endorsed veracity, but only in dealing with other doctors! They didn't mention a need for truth in addressing patients. Doing what was best in the doctor's opinion was not exclusively the arrogance of the medical profession. The moral philosophers of that era agreed completely with the doctors, arguing that lying to a patient in what they perceived to be the best interest of the deceived patient was in fact a virtue. Many cultures today continue to promote that view. The term *informed consent* didn't make its way into medico-legal jargon until 1957, although the need for consent was approached in many earlier legal cases.

For many centuries, beginning in ancient Greece, a single infallible source established ethical behavior in Western culture—the church. In the United States, however, there are many different churches and beliefs. The only thing we have in common is the law, through which we expect equal protection and final resolution of conflicts. That is why the law has played an overriding role in addressing the ethical problems of medicine. The law appears to be congealed ethics. Some judges have been especially articulate in expressing ethical ideas. Of course, not all laws are ethical; we are all familiar with laws that cry out for conscientious violation or civil disobedience, such as those imposing segregation.

But there came a time when legal intercession was desired in a medical case. In 1880, a patient with cataracts sought surgical relief. Being a prudent person, he requested that only one eye be done at a time. Because the surgery was going well, the surgeon did both eyes. Unfortunately, the patient became blind in both eyes, and he sued for malpractice. The surgeon provided witnesses who testified that no negligence had caused the bad outcome, hence there was no malpractice. The issue of consent was not even raised, because what the doctor had done was considered within his discretion. The patient had consented to eye surgery. What type of eye surgery was done was up to the doctor to decide. The case may have ended differently had the patient sued for battery (touching without consent), but he hadn't.

If a patient refused a prescribed medical procedure, it was considered evidence of the patient's incompetence. In one case, a patient accused a surgeon of forcibly chloroforming her and extracting six teeth. His defense was that the surgery was necessary and was performed competently. Besides, in his judgment, the patient lacked the knowledge to judge whether the procedure should have been done. There was a "hung jury," and the doctor went free. The courts left it to the doctor to decide what was in the "best interests" of the patient. That the patient might be best at deciding his or her best interests would have been considered a radical idea.

However, two cases from 1905 and 1906, in Minnesota and Illinois, found that consent was invalid because information had been denied to the patient. One concerned surgery on a patient's ear—the opposite one for which permission had been given. The doctor denied he had operated on the wrong ear, claiming that after the patient was anesthetized, he had reexamined the other ear and determined it was more in need of surgery.

In the second case, the doctor deceived the patient in order to perform a hysterectomy, which she had refused. The operation was done to cure epilepsy—a preposterous theory! This doctor also testified that the disease itself made the patient incompetent to give consent. The patient's husband had assented in order to avoid the need for force. Both cases found for the plaintiff. The decisions spoke of a fundamental right to bodily integrity.

Justice Cardozo, later to be appointed to the U.S. Supreme Court, in a 1914 landmark decision in a New York Court, cited these two cases. Responding to another case in which a surgical procedure was undertaken when consent had been given only to an examination under anesthesia, he wrote, "Every human being of adult years and sound mind has a right to determine what should be done with his own body; and a surgeon who performs an operation without his patient's consent commits an assault."[23]

This was a definite change. It presented the idea that even a necessary and competently performed operation is unacceptable if it is not done with the patient's knowledge and permission.

In 1957, the concept was furthered that for a consent to be considered valid, the patient had to be informed. The plaintiff, paralyzed after aortography (an x-ray with an injection of "dye" into the major artery of the body) complained that he had not been informed that paralysis was a risk of the procedure. The court found that physicians had a duty to disclose the facts that were necessary for a patient to make a decision to undergo or refuse a procedure—the "informed" part of informed consent.[24]

Then in 1960, a Kansas court found that a Dr. Kline had been negligent by not informing a Mrs. Natanson of the possible effects of cobalt radiation for breast cancer. In court, she exposed her chest, permitting each heartbeat to be seen because of destroyed ribs and distention of the overlying skin. Justice Schroeder affirmed the new legal direction by stating, "Anglo-American law starts with the premise of thorough-going self-determination. It follows that each man is master of his own body, and he may, if he be of sound mind, expressly prohibit the performance of life-saving surgery, or other medical treatment."[25]

How has litigation addressed these findings? The doctor is liable for battery if he intervenes without the patient's consent. If the information given is inadequate, negligence is the charge. A standard[26] was established in 1972 that consent ought be based upon what society, rather than the doctor, judges to have been appropriate information for the patient. That lets the jury decide if the information disclosed was adequate for a "reasonable person," to make an informed decision, the jury being presumed to represent "reasonable persons."

The idea that the patient's refusal of a medically beneficial intervention demonstrates his/her incompetence has been abandoned. Some patients have goals in which life and health are not their highest values. This was the case with a Mrs. Candura, a seventy-seven-year-old widow, who in 1978 refused her third partial amputation for gangrene of her feet, which had resulted from advanced diabetes. Her daughter and her doctor went to court in order to obtain legal guardianship so they might force the surgery upon her.

The judge at the appellate level noted she had recently consented to the first two operations. If she had been competent to consent then, why was she now incompetent to refuse? The reply—that she had previously made the right decision—was not acceptable. The judge pointed out that the court was not evaluating the patient's values or the medical appropriateness of the decision, but rather the patient's capacity to make a choice. It was clear that the patient knew her medical condition and the risks and benefits of the procedure, as well as the possible risks (including death) if she refused the procedure. Under these conditions, competent patients must be allowed to make regrettable, even tragic, decisions.[27] This court decision, of course, was the ultimate triumph of the principle of respect for patient autonomy over the principle of beneficence—in other words, upholding a competent patient's self-determined decision instead of complying with whatever the doctor thinks will best promote the patient's health.

To recapitulate, informed consent is necessary to protect patients against harm, intended or not. Consent is necessary to promote their individual interests as they see them, and to promote self-determination, a basic element of our culture. For many centuries, the doctor was expected to act as a parent might be expected to act on behalf of a child. The patient who sought a doctor's ministrations was expected to trust and comply with the doctor's instructions without question. The doctor sought to benefit the patient as he, the doctor (and it was at that time a "he"), interpreted benefit. Whenever the doctor felt deception was in the patient's interest, he would avoid the truth. There was general agreement that engaging a doctor gave him license to treat the patient in whatever way he thought best. A surgeon, given permission to operate, would proceed without discussing details.

As the public grew increasingly more sophisticated, particularly in the United States, more information was demanded and shared with patients. Gradually, as society changed, so did the doctor-patient relationship. Over the past half century, the law moved toward endorsing self-determination, necessarily involving patients in decision making. Patients have to be given sufficient information to participate rationally. It is necessary to be sure that they have the mental capacity for evaluating options and that no coercion is applied. Informed consent is a process, involving discussion with the patient in order to determine and pursue the goals of the patient. Patients must know the alternative choices, along with their risks and benefits, as well as the prognosis if nothing is done. Communication and clarification are essential to the therapeutic relationship. It was the conclusion drawn in the Candura case that I had to apply to Mrs. Wroshaw. Specifically, abiding by a competent patient's self-determined, informed decision—patient-centered medical practice—supersedes what the doctor thinks is the best medical course for the patient.

~

Betty responded to my recommendation that no caesarian be done for fetal distress with a question.

"Would you do that for any other baby—I mean a caesarian—if there were signs that labor was hurting the baby?"

"Well, yes," I replied reluctantly. "I would, but that's different."

"Why is it different?" she replied.

"Because for most other babies—babies without trisomy 18—a caesarian would probably be life-saving, but it's not likely to be for Celeste."

"But might it let her survive labor—and then who knows how long we could have her before she goes to Jesus? Isn't that true?"

Again, there was no gainsaying Betty's speculation. However minimal the benefit appeared to be in *my* mind, in the mind of *Betty* the benefit appeared to be enormous. I thought that whatever the outcome, as a physician, I would not dwell on this event for very long.[28] It would be one of many over a lifetime of practice, I thought, but for Betty—and most probably Ted and Amy—this would be a milestone in their life journey. On balance, if it became necessary— and I fervently hoped it would not—a c-section was only a little more hazardous than a delivery.

I replied, "Yes, that's true."

"Then," asked Betty, "do many babies die in labor? Would it be better to just do a caesarian?"

Ted, who had been silent so far, spoke before I had a chance to answer. "Oh, please don't do that, Betty. I love our baby, but it's not fair to me for you to—to take unnecessary chances. I've gone along because you, well—because you believe so strongly, but I can't believe God wants you to look for trouble. I can't spare you. Amy can't spare you." He appeared distraught, on the verge of a tearful disintegration again.

"All right, Teddy. But you'll let me treat her like any other baby, won't you? I mean, if there were trouble in labor then a caesarian would be right. Okay? Just like any other baby?"

Ted didn't trust himself to speak. He nodded his assent.

"I want to tell you all about c-section, so you understand what your choice would mean," I offered.

We went over the consent issues, including the remote risk of death from surgical complications, and the alternative that I favored—normal vaginal delivery even at the possible sacrifice of Celeste's brief life. To me, surgery would not be a risk that was worth the dubious benefit, but I felt bound to respect their value system. I kept reminding myself that there was no way to rank these competing values, and it was, after all, Betty's baby. Without overwhelming evidence that this was an impermissible choice, I was unable to refuse to do what I had promised her when this tragic possibility had first presented itself.

I recalled a colleague who had promised a Jehovah's Witness that he would not give her a blood transfusion if she should hemorrhage at delivery, even at the risk of her life. It was ironically inevitable that she would be one of the rare cases in his entire career when a patient did have a postpartum hemorrhage. Despite his frantic explanations of her desperate condition, she adamantly refused transfusion, and her husband, standing by, supported her decision. "Better," he said, "to shorten her brief earthly life than to put at risk eternal heavenly life in the arms of Jesus." The patient died despite all the alternative interventions given in lieu of blood. The doctor was devastated. But yearly, on the anniversary of that death, my colleague receives cards of thanks from the patient's husband and many of his friends from the Witness community. People hold strong opinions in such cases, but no one asserts there is incontrovertible proof of who is right.

ᔕ

Betty went into labor conveniently for both of us, at five in the morning, about two weeks before her due date—not unexpected for a second baby. When I came to the labor deck, I explained the situation to the nurses and residents on call. I also told them of her choice regarding a c-section, because I expected there would be fetal distress. Some of them had not encountered a trisomy 18 before, so we had a brief refresher course. One of the residents showed his disapproval by voicing more a statement than a question, "You're going to put a scar on the uterus for a baby that's unlikely to live more than a few hours?" His concern was for the risk should the mother become pregnant again. There was danger of internal rupture of the uterine scar and hemorrhage. Babies rarely survived such a catastrophe, and mothers frequently had a close call. Some doctors recommended "once a section, always a section."

"I would prefer not to," I said, "but if you knew this lady, you'd know there would be a far worse scar on her mind and psyche if we didn't do a section—if we found evidence of fetal distress."

The resident looked skeptical, but in deference to my experience, or perhaps more in deference to my position relative to his, he said no more. I told him we should get together at lunch and talk about obstetrics, autonomy, and theology a while. He didn't look reassured.

Some patients, knowing their fetus has a severe anomaly, refuse monitoring to avoid the decision they would have to make if distress is noted. Betty had asked to be monitored. I made rounds, checked in with her again as she progressed in early labor, then went to my office across the street, expecting a call momentarily. I was not disappointed, although I would have preferred to have been. Problems with the heartbeat were registered, and meconium[29] had appeared. I gave instructions over the phone to prepare for a section, and Betty was in the operating room by the time I had arrived and changed my clothes. Just as we had her washed and draped, and epidural anesthesia had been placed, the pediatrician arrived. He had been thoroughly oriented by Betty and me several weeks before. He had explained to Betty and Ted that he did not intend to be very aggressive. When babies are born very ill, he told them, he believed they should be kept warm, kept free of any obstruction to breathing, and then observed—in his words, "to see if they want to live." That was agreeable to the Wroshaws. They didn't want their baby to be subjected to painful interventions if they would almost certainly be futile.

The surgery went quickly and the baby was delivered uneventfully. I placed her in the bassinet, but I could see she was limp and not yet breathing. I left her in the hands of the pediatrician and turned back to Betty to await the afterbirth and begin closing the wound. Betty could look over at the pediatrician, who I assumed was trying to stimulate the baby to cry. I heard a tiny whimper and didn't know whether I was relieved or not. I guess it's intuitive for all of us to push for life, even a truncated life.

Ted had been permitted to sit above the ether screen at the level of Betty's head. The pediatrician brought Celeste wrapped in a warm blanket over to Ted, who held her. Betty reached out to touch her, smiling broadly even as tears rolled down her cheeks. "I forgot how tiny they are," she said. Celeste was not crying, but she was breathing shallowly.

"I'm going to take her to the nursery now to clean her up and do a quick exam," the pediatrician said, "and by the time you get to OB recovery, I'll bring her back." Betty appeared as if she didn't want to part with her baby for a minute, but she agreed to that brief separation.

When the pediatrician brought her back, Celeste still had the blue tint of a newborn. This coloring results when the circulating blood has less than normal oxygen levels. That's normal inside the womb, but outside, when a baby is breathing with normal lungs and the blood is circulated by an efficiently pumping heart, the blood is red and the baby becomes pink. This process wasn't happening for Celeste.

Although Betty exclaimed, "Isn't she beautiful!" it was apparent to objective eyes that many of Celeste's features were aberrant. Her head was small in proportion to her body, the ears were low set and somewhat pointed on top. Both eyes were narrow and her mouth was small. She was cute in an elfin-like way, but clearly unusual in appearance. The malformed hands and feet seen in the ultrasound were just as we had described them at that time. Breathing was labored. I peeked under the blanket and saw a large protrusion where the navel should have been, with intestine bulging against a sac. I guessed the pediatrician had found the baby so nearly dying that he brought her out so she could spend her last minutes, or maybe a few hours, with her mother and father.

As he handed the baby over to Betty, the pediatrician said, "I'm so sorry, but the baby has such severe heart and lung problems that we can't do anything to save her. I thought it would be better for her to be with you here than in the nursery. I truly believe she will stop breathing soon."

Betty reached out for Celeste and brought her to lie on her chest. "Thank you for telling the truth and being so thoughtful, Doctor." She turned to Ted and said, "Can you take some pictures?" Then as a quick follow-up, she said, "And as soon as you do, would you get Mom and Amy from the waiting room? That's okay, isn't it, Doctor?" she asked, turning to me.

This was certainly the time to ignore hospital rules about recovery room visitors. There was no telling how long the baby would live, and the one remaining grandmother and the soon-to-be-disappointed big sister should have a chance to say hello before a sad goodbye.

"Certainly," I said.

As the remaining family members arrived, I greeted them and told everyone I was leaving for my office but would return on evening rounds. Later that day when I returned, I stopped at the nurse's station to learn what had transpired. The baby had died about four in the afternoon in her mother's arms. As I took a deep breath and stepped into the room, I saw the close family members were still there. Much to my surprise, eyes were dry. Amy had crayons and a large notepad. She was busily drawing what I soon deciphered to be her baby sister with wings, hovering around a sheeted figure with a halo.

"You've heard?" asked Betty.

"Yes," I replied. "I'm so sorry things couldn't have turned out better."

"Well, now Celeste has a perfect body and is in the loving arms of Jesus forever," she told me. "No one could ask for more."

"And we'll all be together in heaven someday," piped up Amy.

❧

Betty's physical recovery was quick. We spoke lengthily on rounds. She told me not to be fooled by her apparent equanimity—that she was hurting a good deal inside but knew Celeste was in a better world, and that enabled her to be at peace with the events of the past year.

Then she told me she was holding Celeste when her soul left her. She felt a physical difference as it went, she said. "I know you're a skeptic," she continued, "but I want you to know that the two hours we spent together with the baby were extremely precious to all of us. I thank God for giving us those treasured moments. We will cherish them all our lives. And I thank you for not getting in the way."

I felt a little awkward, and all I could think to say was, "How is Ted doing? I have missed him on rounds."

"He must be doing well, Doctor. He asked me to ask you what the chances were for this happening when we became pregnant again."

I loved the way she said "when *we* became pregnant again." I told her the statistics were one in a hundred or less for a recurrence of trisomy 18.

"Well, I'm not quite ready to try again, but it isn't out of the question. Let's see how soon I get back in shape. I don't want to do it too soon, because I don't want people to think I'm trying to replace Celeste. That can't ever be done. She'll always be in my heart."

Soon after, Betty went home. I saw her post-op and removed the staples. The wound healed well. After she dressed and returned to my consultation room, she said, "You know, I hadn't recovered enough to go to the funeral, so we announced that we would have a memorial service instead. It would be nice if you could come."

"When is it?" I asked.

"Next Tuesday morning," she replied, "at eleven."

"I'm truly sorry, but I have surgery scheduled and I really can't postpone it."

"I understand."

"Will you send me the program and pretend I was there?" I asked.

"Of course I will, and I'll always be grateful that you thought enough of me to go against your medical judgment and do what in my heart I knew was the right thing for Celeste. I know she's with her heavenly father right now, and she too is grateful for the chance to have had a brief life with me, Ted, Amy, and my mother."

In the newspaper the next day, there was a notice of a memorial service with the time, date, and location. At the head of the column was a picture. It showed the diminutive face of Celeste snuggled in a little hospital cap. The column underneath said, "Two weeks ago, Celeste Wroshaw had a brief visit with her mommy, Betty, her daddy, Ted, her big sister, Amy, and her grandma before she went on to eternal life in the arms of her Heavenly Father. Please join us for prayers of thanks and rejoicing for the chance we were given to spend time with our beautiful daughter before she became a beautiful angel."

♪

When I ruminate about patients of deep faith who I have encountered in my practice, other patients who have confronted tribulation such as Betty Wroshaw's, it has become clear to me that their faith does not protect them from the pain of tragedy—pain that we will all experience in our lifetimes. However, it surely provides them with a buttress that they may lean upon at such times, and it sustains them until the storms pass. Such a gift is enviable.

BLACK AND WHITE

Life is easier for people who think philosophically in terms of black or white. The troubling shades of gray confound the rest of us. The difficulty I encountered this day concerned the thorniest of problems—abortion. I won't rehash the numerous arguments that you've probably heard and read, but I will touch briefly on some that are relevant to my narrative.

There are those who believe that the moment a sperm penetrates an egg, the resultant embryo is a person entitled to all the legal and moral rights accorded a competent adult. There is no doubt that in the right environment, the embryo is capable of self-directed continuous development with the potential to become a person. But others maintain that, although the genetic makeup of the embryo is unquestionably human, it is not enough to consider this structure equal to a child or adult. They hold that this is not a human being, but rather a human *becoming*. They assert that there is more to being a human, to personhood—things like being able to feel, and having some level of consciousness and some recognizable form. They compare an embryo to a depot that holds building materials within that are not yet a house.

There are contradictions in these arguments because, if self-consciousness or reasoning were required to define the status of personhood, infants—like embryos—wouldn't qualify for protection. And if entry to the right to life is sentience or feeling, then animals *do* have this right. But most people believe newborn infants possess a right to life and that animals don't necessarily possess this right. So, the presence or absence of these faculties apparently doesn't serve adequately to separate embryos from other human entities. Of course, some who don't feel embryos have the standing of persons maintain that the embryo is simply too immature a form of human life to merit the protection that we provide more-developed humans. However, if nothing is established that unquestionably identifies the stage of human development after which destroying a human life is morally wrong, it's reasonable to assert that it is wrong to destroy any embryo.

The fertilized egg is called a zygote that, with cell division, becomes an embryo. Then, at eight weeks of gestation, it is called a fetus until birth. Not everyone who is opposed to abortion maintains that the fertilized egg has an unquestionable right to life. Many feel that abortion should be permitted, for example, to save the mother's life. But to be consistent, when a woman knowingly risks a pregnancy, anyone who truly regards the fetus as a person should argue that the innocent fetus should take precedence over the risk-taking woman. However, few hold that position, and most people feel a mother is justified in aborting a fetus when it is a matter of self-defense. Yet this position is inconsistent with the belief that a fetus is a person with an incontrovertible right to live.

Few people believe that it is justifiable for a third party, even a doctor, to kill an innocent person to save another, but many who oppose abortion find it permissible when pregnancy is the result of rape or incest, even though the pregnancy is the result of a crime of which the fetus is also innocent. The fact that people make these exceptions suggest there is some common ground between liberal and conservative views on destroying embryos. The implication is that early forms of human life can sometimes be sacrificed. Some very influential conservatives accept that it is permissible to destroy embryos when it is necessary to save lives or preserve health. This presumably is the position of anti-abortion advocates who nevertheless support stem cell research. On precisely what grounds they decide that there is greater value to the interests of adult humans than to the interests of the fetus or embryo is uncertain. But liberals and some conservatives agree that the destruction of embryos is permissible where there is good reason to believe that it is necessary to preserve life or restore a severely compromised quality of life. And, more to the point of this story, some reach even further, finding it permissible to terminate for its own sake the life of a fetus that at birth will be doomed by severe abnormalities to either a brief or painfully prolonged life of suffering.

⌒

On the day of this narrative, I was confronted by a black-and-white problem in every sense of the word. I was making evening rounds later than usual, about seven thirty in the evening, when a nurse appeared at the nurse's station where I was writing my notes in the charts. Apparently, she was looking for a specific physician, but it seems the other attending physicians that day had already been able to finish up and go home. No one else was there except a nurse's aide.

"Dr. Abrams, I know this isn't your patient, but I'm really having trouble in 336," she said apologetically.

"What's wrong?"

"Well, Janelle McCormick is here for a D & E first thing in the morning, and her boyfriend is in there trying to force her to leave. He said if she doesn't come with him, he's going to drag her out, and he actually pushed me out of the room."

⌒

The vast majority of abortions are done at less than twelve weeks of pregnancy by suction curettage, termed a D & C (dilation and curettage). Tissue, usually unrecognizable, is removed by using a narrow suction tube, often less than a half inch in diameter. Another procedure, called a D & E (dilation and evacuation) is hospital terminology for an abortion that's done when the pregnancy is beyond the first twelve weeks, often fourteen or sixteen weeks, rarely more. Only a few doctors did D & Es, because it's emotionally difficult for everyone involved. Despite its small size, the fetus has a recognizable form. For the pregnant patient, it is not safe to remove it without enlarging the opening to the uterus, called the cervix.

In the late 1960s and 1970s, early in the history of legal abortions, the safety of D & E as an outpatient procedure had not yet been established. Patients were admitted the night before, and a device was inserted into the cervix to prepare it for surgery. How it was ever discovered that a twig-like segment of seaweed had just the right characteristics to slowly swell overnight and painlessly enlarge the uterine opening, I daren't even speculate. Nevertheless, this organic object, alien to the animal body, properly sterilized and packaged, became a standard part of surgical procedures calling for dilation of the cervix. This process minimized the risk of injuring the tissue when it had to be opened wide enough to empty the uterus. And of great importance, once the dilation process was begun, was that there was no turning back without significant risk to both mother and fetus. The cervix is a barrier to outside microorganisms that can cause infection. Opening it exposes the susceptible uterus to infection, with potentially serious consequences to the patient. The hazard increases the longer the cervix remains open.

⁓

There wasn't much time to probe the details of the patient's history as I was enroute to her room, or the reason for a second-trimester abortion. I asked the aide to call security stat and hastened toward room 336, asking the nurse if she knew why the abortion was being done. She told me it was because the patient had contracted rubella from her younger sister during her first month of pregnancy.

Rubella is known by common terminology as German measles. Ordinarily, it's a mild disease characterized by a rash and fever. Three-quarters of the American population has contracted it before they reach reproductive age, but for those who haven't, it constitutes a serious threat to pregnancy. Significant fetal abnormalities occur in half the babies born if rubella is contracted in the first month of pregnancy. The problems vary from fetal deafness to fetal death in the uterus. Fetal brain infection can be a cause of retardation later if the fetus survives. Heart malformations and bleeding tendencies have also been attributed to fetal infection with the virus in the first sixteen weeks of pregnancy. Most doctors will offer termination of pregnancy for confirmed cases of rubella in early pregnancy. I suspected that was the reason why this one was being done.

I walked into the room and saw a young black man who appeared to be in his twenties standing by the bed and tightly gripping the patient's outstretched arm at the wrist. His T-shirt, which was tucked into jeans at a wide-belted tapered waist, revealed a dauntingly muscular torso. While I was contemplating what in heck I had gotten myself into, he took the initiative.

"What you lookin' at, honky?"

Collecting my thoughts quickly, and inspired by an instinct for self-preservation, I replied, "I'm looking at a man who I bet has good intentions, but he's assaulted a nurse and, whether he knows it or not, is about to endanger this young lady's life. Now let her go, and let's talk about it before you get arrested and put yourself in deep shit."

Maybe because he didn't expect profanity (albeit mild) from a man in a white coat, but for whatever reason, and to my everlasting surprise and satisfaction, he released her arm and turned to me. When I saw that he didn't intend to go after me—at least at that moment— I continued. "I'm not sure you know about what's going on here."

"Dam straight I do. Yoo bassards make a pile a money and kill off us 'lousy niggers' at the same time and it ain't nothing to yoo."

"Wait a second, do you know why she's here?"

"I just tol' ya, din I, now les go," he said, turning to the girl.

She scooted further away to the far side of her bed. "I ain' goin' nowhere wit yoo. How come you got so inerested now, when I'm inna hospital but you was nowhere when I aks you before?"

I was glad to see he had simmered down enough to talk, but I thought it would be nice to see the security guard show up. "Wait a second. Do you know she caught German measles from her kid sister?"

"No—so what? German measles ain' no big deal. I had 'em."

She broke in, turning to me. "It ain' oney the German measles, 'cause 'fore I knew what it was, I tol' him I was pregnant and I wanneda get married 'n' he tol' me to screw off." She turned back to him, "Din ya?"

"Not bein' married ain' no reason to kill off another black baby," he retorted. "Ya jus' playin' the white man's game. What you think all them Planned Parenthood clinics are doin' in Five Points, anyway? You don' see 'em inna fancy neighborhoods, do ya?"

I jumped back in. "Hey, you can think whatever you want to, but right now, things have gone too far here to go back. This young lady has started treatment, and two things will happen if she leaves. First, she's at a big risk for infection unless this is finished up by tomorrow. Second, she's likely to go on and miscarry by herself anyway, although it would take a few days and hurt like hell, and then she's even more likely to get an infection that could kill her."

There was some uncertainty in his voice when he declared, "Ya jus' sayin' that, man." Then, with even less conviction, turning away, "Ya don' give a shit."

"No, I'm not just saying that. And you don't know what German measles can do to babies. She had it early when she got pregnant, so there's a fifty-fifty chance of heart disease or brain damage or deafness and lots of other nasty things. That's why she found a doctor that would do an abortion past the usual time. And it's her choice, you know. It's something you might have chosen, too, right along with her if you'd have gotten involved when she asked you—if you'd stayed around long enough to know a little more about what could happen."

Security arrived in the person of a uniformed guard, and I was glad to see he was black. He asked, "What's going on?"

He addressed the guard, "Nothin'. Anyway, yoo got the gun. Okay, Uncle Tom, I'm goin'." He turned to the girl. "But I ain' finished wit yoo."

I couldn't tell from the way he said it whether it was a threat or an apology. He left the room, and the guard strode after him, saying, "I'll see you to the door."

After he had gone, it was hard to concentrate on finishing my charts. I was still buzzing with adrenaline, and my thoughts wouldn't settle down. I thought how different this young man's outlook was from that of the brilliant black pathologist whom I had heard lecture at the medical school a few weeks ago—or was it different? Had that doctor, or another of my patients, an articulate black historian/schoolteacher, or the black receptionist in my colleague's office, overcome the same or different barriers? Had they learned the language differently or had the young man simply chosen to speak "black" in defiance of the world he perceived as oppressive to him and his race? Was it a reflection of race or economic class that made him different from the blacks among my professional contacts—the black surgeon, for example, whom I had chosen to operate on my wife? If that was so, was his early upbringing one of poverty or opportunity never offered? Had he perhaps suffered an experience early in life that had colored his outlook ineradicably from that point on? For a long time, I've been aware that blacks are suspicious of the predominately white medical establishment. I know from old medical records and journal reports that blacks were mistreated by doctors when, as slaves, they were denied treatment at the whim of masters who did not wish to invest in a worn-out "property." As slaves also, they were subjected to atrocious experiments as unconsenting research subjects, and as free men they were similarly deceived into the 1970s and beyond.[30]

I'm aware that, as a group, blacks continue to be underdiagnosed and undertreated. Their mortality is greater from the same illnesses, and the fetal death rate is higher than it is in whites. I had hoped that, with the maturing of the civil rights movement, some trust from the black community had been earned by doctors who worked pro bono poor black communities. I had hoped that eloquent words asking whites to make America "a nation where they will not be judged by the color of their skin but by the content of their character," might also appeal to young black men so they did not grow up believing all whites were the enemy.

I'm not sure whether the arrival of an armed guard had made it possible for the young black man to leave and save face or if he left because he actually believed what I had said about rubella and the danger to her if she left the hospital. I'm still haunted by his genuine conviction that a white conspiracy exists, an organized movement to kill off blacks, and that doctors were playing a deliberate role in geno-cide by performing abortions. We have a long way to go with race in the United States, don't we?

THEY SHOOT HORSES

I was alarmed when I saw Norma Radwell for her annual GYN exam. It was as if she were a different person from the healthy woman in her late forties who I had seen just the year before. I had first met her when she became a new patient. She had moved to town a few months before that first visit a year ago, from the West Coast with her husband, Lane, and her only child, Bobby.

She had remained in my memory very vividly because she had been so agitated. I remembered the dreadfully disturbing experience that she told me had happened on the very day of her appointment. Of course, I knew that many women are uncomfortable visiting any gynecologist, especially a new one, particularly if they shared with their previous doctor the experience of childbirth. But it appeared to be more than that. When I saw her in the waiting room, she was picking distractedly at threads on her knobby tweed coat, deeply preoccupied with her thoughts. She was startled when I called her name, jumping a little in the straight-backed chair she had chosen. After I had guided her into my office from the waiting room and had introduced myself, I offered, "You look a little upset, Mrs. Radwell. (She actually looked more than "a little" distressed.) I hope we haven't done anything to upset you. We're only running five minutes behind."

"Oh, no," she replied. "It's nothing here, no." She paused. "But you're right." She looked down at her hands in her lap and her voice trembled. "I almost didn't come in today."

"Do you want to tell me what's wrong?" I asked.

She bit her lower lip and looked through me to some vision she was re-creating. Her eyes misted, and she said, "I don't know if I can. It was so awful."

I waited.

She looked at me and asked, "Do you have any pets?"

"Not any more," I said, "but I had a wonderful dog when I was growing up."

"Then maybe you'll understand. I love horses, and I've always ridden several times a week." Then she looked at me a little more intensely, cocked her head, and asked, "Do you have time to listen to this?"

"Of course," I replied, which was a white lie.

Norma quickly filled in her history. She was a CPA, and in California she had specialized in preparing tax returns. In her spare time, she had become an accomplished equestrian and had many ribbons to show for it. After she had become pregnant with Bobby, she and her husband had talked it over and decided that motherhood was a full-time job, at least until Bobby went off to school. For a few years, raising Bobby was enough for her. Then she had managed to combine caring for her home and family—especially the oversight of her growing boy—with part-time tax preparation, and she contentedly watched the years go by.

Then her husband came home one evening and, after dinner, told her his company had offered him a promotion and a substantial raise, provided they would move to Colorado. They talked it over and decided that, despite California attachments, it was a very good offer and the opportunity overrode the objections. Besides, they had enjoyed dude ranching in Colorado for many summers. Living in Colorado would provide a chance for Norma to ride in open country, which she liked best of all. They found the respite each summer from crowded Los Angeles a welcome change. So, off they went to a new adventure; Lane looked forward to conquering new worlds in business, and Norma anticipated the opportunity to foster her enjoyment of horses.

Once the turmoil of relocation was completed, Norma found an opening in a large accounting firm and resumed part-time work.

Bobby had transferred to a Colorado college to continue his engineering studies. Although he came home frequently, he lived at school and did not add significantly to Norma's housekeeping chores.

She had continued her regular exercise program, riding horseback two or three times a week and also jogging in the early evening—sometimes with Bobby, when he was home, and sometimes with Lane, after the dinner and dishes were done.

Norma continued, "Today was a riding day, and I usually start very early and finish by noon so I can do my other things in the afternoon. I drove out on I-225 toward Bailey, where there's this resort that has a great stable, and rode Piebald. She's my favorite. We had a wonderful ride. The air was crisp and the aspen are in full color, and of course, the sky was that wonderful clear blue we love here—not a cloud. I was heading back and we were close to the stable when I saw smoke coming from right where we were going. We slowed down because we could see it was actually coming from the stable."

Here Norma stopped, and once again, her eyes took on a glazed appearance as she conjured up a vision of what had transpired. "When we got there, there was a group of people around a horse lying on the ground and a lot of yelling, but the awful thing was the horse. It was writhing around and screaming. I mean I never heard such a noise—a noise like that—from a horse. Its head was all burnt, and it had no lips—it was horrible. And it wouldn't stop." Her voice dropped. "It wouldn't stop."

Norma was shaking now and crying, and the only thing I could do was grab a handful of tissues from my desk and hold them out to her. There were no words that came to me. She bunched up the tissues and dabbed her eyes. I suspect she had lost any notion of her current surroundings as she looked at the scene in her mind's eye.

"Then," she said, "the wrangler came running up and he had a gun, and he came around from the horse's back so he wouldn't be kicked, and the horse was just thrashing around and the wrangler put it to his head and shot him. And I thought how hard and how sad it was for the wrangler to kill his horse that he probably loved and how merciful to put him out of his agony."

Then she slowly came back into the present and, continuing to weep silently, said, "I'm sorry. It was just so terrible. Somebody had spilled a container of gasoline from the tractor right next to the stall; somehow it splashed over him and then something must have set it off—a spark or something. And then I drove home, and I haven't had a chance to tell anyone about it until you." She smiled wryly through the tears and said, "So I unloaded on you and I'm sorry."

I had unconsciously been holding my breath, and I let it out with a whoosh as I answered, "Well, I'm glad you had a chance to tell somebody. I think the more you talk about it—sort of air it out—the sooner you'll polish off the jagged edges. You're not going to forget it—that's not what I mean—but it won't be so disruptive for you. So don't hold back, and don't be embarrassed about talking to me about it. It was a terrible experience. You need to talk about it."

She did a few final dabs with the tissues and then said, "I guess I'm ready for my exam now. I filled out my papers. Was there anything more you need to know?"

After the exam was completed, I remarked on her good physical condition and especially on how young and healthy she appeared; she showed no signs of menopause, which might be beginning in many of her contemporaries as they approached fifty. I had had no advice to offer her except to remember the annual mammograms and pap smears and to come see me in a year, or whenever she felt like it. I couldn't help but add, "and get back on the horse," as if she had had a fall.

⌇

But today, only a year later, there was a disturbing difference—enough for me to dispense with the usual opening pleasantries and to say, "Mrs. Radwell, you are looking pale and you are quite thin compared to last year. What's going on?"

"Well, you're right. I didn't want to become one of those menopausal whiners, so I've been ignoring my symptoms until I just couldn't anymore."

"Tell me about it."

"Well, it's hard to say when it started; I think it's been about a year, maybe just after my visit here. It didn't come on all at once. I noticed I woke up stiff every morning. I thought it was from my regular evening jog. But it seemed to be lasting longer and longer—the stiffness, I mean. And when I was cleaning up the house, if I stopped to rest, I was stiff again when I got up. Even though I was resting more often, it didn't seem to help." She frowned. "I was getting depressed, especially when I felt hot and I figured that this was the beginning of hot flushes, and I'm getting to be an old lady. My husband noticed I wasn't eating much, and it was obvious I was letting him and Bobbie jog without me, so he asked me what was wrong. I didn't want to be one of those complaining housewives on TV, so I didn't say much about the stiffness. I just told him I was tired and I figured I was low on estrogen, but," she explained, looking up at me, "you had said when you checked me that everything looked normal, so I didn't want to come back so soon."

Norma went on. "Then they got better, the aches and pains, and I felt pretty good for a while. I even started riding again. I thought I might be better from some herbs I found for menopause. But it came back again after a few weeks. The clincher was something that happened two weeks ago." Holding up both hands, she demonstrated. "My fingers swelled up on both hands. Even vacuuming made my wrists sore. So, am I in menopause? Do I need hormones?"

"Tell me, are you menstruating regularly?"

"Yes, but they're not as heavy."

I continued, "But they're on time and you haven't skipped any?"

She caught the hint of skepticism in my questions. "That's right, but can't it be menopause anyway?" She sounded as if she hoped it was menopause. "What about the flushes?"

"Well, are they really flushes, or do you think you may have had a little fever? Did your face get red?"

"No—well, maybe a little flushed—but it kind of stays that way when I'm warm. They don't come and go. What else could it be?"

"Let's do our exam and then I may be a little smarter."

I did the routine GYN physical, noted the normal breast exam and the confirming mammogram report, and did the pelvic and paps. But this time, I deviated from a strictly GYN exam and paid special attention to the fingers and hands. The knuckles were swollen and sore, and the next joint up, the fingers were diffusely swollen and red. The outsides of the wrists also were very tender. "Okay, let's go to my office and talk."

Norma looked worried, and I suspect she had caught my expression. Sometimes I can't keep a poker face unless I concentrate on it. "So," she asked, frowning, "what do you think? Is it early menopause?"

"I don't think so. Tissues look well estrogenized. I mean, you don't appear to have any lack of hormones."

"So then, what?"

"It looks like arthritis."

"Is that all?" she sighed with relief. "That's not a big deal. Lane had some in his shoulder, and he took ibuprofen and felt okay again. So do you think some of those NSAIDS (nonsteroidal anti-inflammatory drugs) will fix it?"

"Well, Norma, let me explain. There are different kinds of arthritis. Sounds like Lane had osteoarthritis. He kind of wore out the cartilage in his shoulder joint. That will often respond to NSAIDS and local treatment, like heating pads."

"So, won't I?"

"Well, I would guess you have a different kind that doesn't clear up so easily."

"What do you mean—'doesn't clear up so easily'?"

"Norma, I'm a GYN and that's beyond me—the details, I mean. But I know when someone ought to see an expert, and I'd like to refer you to one, a rheumatologist who knows all there is to know about joints and muscles and the things that you're complaining about."

Norma ruminated a moment and then said, "At least you're not sending me to a shrink. You don't think it's all in my head, do you?"

"No, Norma, it's not, and they're not the kind of symptoms that come from estrogen deficiency—from menopause. So let's get you hooked up with a good rheumatologist, and soon. I'll call him now if it's okay with you."

I arranged an appointment for Norma with Roy Williams, a bright and sympathetic specialist. After many years of internal medicine practice, he had gone into rheumatology, the specialty associated with joints and muscles and the tissues that connect all the supportive structures of the body.

A few weeks after Norma's visit, I received a report from Roy. He confirmed my guess. Indeed, Norma had rheumatoid arthritis, and it had come on rapidly. Blood tests confirmed it, and x-rays already showed thinning in the bones around her joints. He went on to explain some of the treatment he planned to use. I learned that the potent and sometimes toxic medications, which he had to monitor carefully, were in categories so wordy that he used the first letters of the group to refer to them. He gave me examples, which sometimes were more than I wanted to remember, words such as NSAIDS and the potent DMARDS, disease-modifying antirheumatic drugs.

He wrote that he would be following Norma closely, with frequent testing, because these medications have many side effects. It would be wise, he suggested, for me to also ask about symptoms when I saw her for her GYN exams, because checking for visual changes, ulcers with bleeding, and signs of heart and kidney failure couldn't be done too frequently. These complications, we both knew, are relatively rare, but clearly they are quite serious. The effects of the disease are so devastating when they are allowed to progress that such potentially deadly medications were acceptable, when one is balancing the risks.

I saw Norma almost yearly after that, when she returned for her annual exam. What I saw was very disheartening. She took medicines to combat the disease and medicines to combat the effects of those medicines. She had to give up jogging because similar pain and swelling began in her feet. Horseback riding was long since abandoned. She was having difficulty even doing housework. As a decade went by, it was apparent that she had one of the most severe cases of rheumatoid arthritis I had ever seen. She had gone from needing special tools to put on stockings, open jars, and hold a pen to the point she could be helped only by surgery. At first, the operations were relatively minor, on her feet so she could walk; then they progressed to knee and hip replacements. Now and again, she had skipped examinations with me because of incapacity that came and went, but mostly came.

Throughout all of this destructive illness, Lane had been a staunch ally against despair and reclusiveness. When necessary—and it wasn't always; she had good periods as well as bad—he pushed her in her wheelchair, helped with toileting, and made sure to take her out to movies and social events. They had hired daytime help. Bobby had married but remained as close as a son could be, although he was understandably quite occupied with a busy work schedule and two small children. Bobby's wife and Norma had a courteous relationship, pleasant enough, but far from the bonding that can develop when a family is lucky enough to incorporate a warm mother-daughter connection. The grandchildren were a source of great pleasure when they visited, but at the same time they were rather wearing on Grandma.

Then catastrophe was heaped upon tragedy. Lane died suddenly. He was only sixty-two when he had a heart attack at work that did not respond to resuscitative efforts. Their primary care doctor worked in the same building as I did, and he told me in the parking lot. My first comment wasn't, "Poor Lane." Instead, I blurted out, "Poor Norma." This was not the expected turn of events. It was the wrong sequence. Norma had an illness that shortened life expectancy, not Lane. Really, he had been her lifeline—her connection to the world. He was the agent who facilitated the events that allowed her to get the most out of her life, despite her limited mobility and pain.

Her grief and depression were profound. Her primary care doctor placed her on antidepressant medication. She continued on one or another of them indefinitely. Bobby and the children spent more time with her, and he offered her a room at his house, She refused, however, not wishing to add her burden to his already overloaded schedule. It was about two years after Lane's death that I received a phone call from Roy at home in the evening. I hadn't seen Norma since Lane died.

"Hi, Fred, you know Norma Radwell, don't you?" He paused. "Of course! You referred her to me, didn't you? Anyway, recently she's had a bout with vasculitis."

"I'm not sure what that means, Roy. I mean, I know the terminology, but what are her symptoms?"

"She's losing weight again, but that's not so bad. It's the other things going wrong with the blood vessels that worry me, and a steroid boost that usually helps so quickly isn't doing much for her. Her eyes are red and painful and they're sensitive to light. She's having trouble seeing, so she has even more problems getting around. She can walk better since she got new knees, but the pain from her toes limits her. But the most distressing symptoms now are new ulcers from blocked blood vessels on both of her legs, some toes, and her index finger on her right hand. They all hurt, and all indications are that it's going to get worse. She's loaded with pain meds, so she's groggy, too. What's more, those ulcers can get infected, and if the vasculitis becomes really widespread, it can cause stroke or heart failure.

"What a miserable disease!"

"Yeah. She's pretty bad. Hey, you ran that conference on suicide, didn't you?"

"Yes, in '86."

"Was it about helping or preventing?"

"Actually both. We had speakers who work to prevent suicide, like with teenagers or depressed patients. We had speakers who advocated PAS [physician-assisted suicide] for terminal patients."

"The guy who founded the Hemlock Society was there, right?"

"Yes." I wasn't sure where Roy was going with this, so I just waited.

"He's written books on this, hasn't he? Do you have any?"

"Sure I do and lots of other books, too. So what's on your mind, Roy?"

"Well, today Norma asked me the sixty-four-thousand-dollar question."

"Yes?"

"Last week, she had the last digit of a toe amputated—it was gangrenous because the vasculitis had stopped the blood supply. She said she wanted to talk seriously with me and to set some extra time aside. We sat down in my office, and I'll try to go over what she said. She started out with, 'I've got a lot to talk about and I want to start with this. I don't do well without my husband. I miss the companionship, and to be really honest, I miss the intimacy. A person needs touching. We knew that one of us might end up taking care of the other, and that was all right with us. It turned out he drew the short straw, or maybe I did. But I believe having to take care of a sick person is harder than being sick, so I think he had the bigger burden. Lots of people my age go out and find somebody to be a companion after one of them dies,' she went on, 'but we had a bond because of my illness that was unique, and we made the best of it. I don't think I'd look for anybody even if I could, but,' she smiled ruefully, 'I can't exactly go to the nearest singles bar. Now, on top of that, the last straw. I've got this damned painful vasculitis that never stops, and I'm beginning to be whittled on, and I don't see any end to it. This is not a life. I can see me stuck in some hospital somewhere full of tubes and needles, not sick enough to die and not well enough to live. I don't want that.'"

Roy paused and then said, "Fred, that's about it, but the bottom line is, she wants to commit suicide and she wants me to help."

Somewhere in the United States, doctors confront the issue of physician-assisted suicide every day, but I hadn't yet encountered it in one of my patients. Of course, Dr. Williams was managing the main problem for Mrs. Radwell, but I still felt involved.

~

There's widespread debate about how far a doctor can go. Generally, it's fair to say that doctors must be devoted to life and health. But individual patients aren't interested in life and health as abstractions. Rather, they're devoted to specific desires about their own life and health, and they expect the physician to apply medical skills to achieve their goals. What happens if the patient determines that a time has come when death is preferable to life?

Physicians work with the objective to produce the best medical outcome for the patient, in keeping with agreed-upon objectives. It is a dynamic relationship with changing goals and interventions as the course of an illness unfolds. Sometimes, a cure is not possible and the caring aspects of the relationship become the focus. Certainly, that's true with a chronic and disabling disease like rheumatoid arthritis.

Few people deny any longer that a person may refuse any medical treatment, including life-sustaining treatment. Aside from the ethical consensus, the U.S. Supreme Court affirmed the legality of refusal in the Cruzan case more than a decade ago.[31] No change in the law would be necessary for Norma to die by refusing nutrition and hydration, as established by an advance directive, if she were comatose. However, Norma's situation was compounded by the fact that she did not have a terminal illness. To be sure, it is a nasty illness, but unless something more drastic happened, she was no more terminal than most other patients in their early sixties. A profound change in the law would be necessary for Dr. Williams to provide the means for suicide by supplying a lethal prescription. If doctors acted upon what they felt was a moral duty to comply with a patient's request for a lethal dose of medication, in any state but Oregon a physician would be criminally liable.

Some people, including some mental health experts, assert that suicide is always irrational. Many religious systems find suicide to be unacceptable on the basis that a person's life is held in trust, given by God and to be taken only by God. This is a decision based on faith, and for those who have that faith, it may serve them well. But many persons, religious and otherwise, agree that there are circumstances of unbearable suffering that justify suicide, and that this choice ought to be available to patients for whom suffering plays no redemptive role in their philosophy.

If they had ready access to lethal medications, such patients would not have to call upon physicians for prescriptions. In the United States, these drugs are not available by any legitimate means except in the state of Oregon. I have heard people say, "Well, anybody can go to the street and get whatever they want." That response is simply a cruel evasion, particularly if it is addressed, for example, to a virtually immobile patient with a cancer metastatic to the spine, or one paralyzed with amyotrophic lateral sclerosis (Lou Gehrig's disease, or ALS), or one drowning in secretions from a widely invasive cancer of the tongue or larynx.

Physicians are licensed by society to dispense medications, providing checks and balances against ill-considered or impulsive acts by patients. Some persons argue that if there were a method by which a desperate patient might approach their physician for aid-in-dying, some lives could be saved rather than lost. Patients who misunderstood a diagnosis or prognosis, those who were depressed and who might respond to treatment, or those who simply needed to know that someone supported them in their difficulty might be persuaded to forbear. However, once a doctor is satisfied that temporary depression, misinformation, or misunderstanding play no role in a competent patient's decision, he may relinquish the paternalistic role and enable his patient to bypass the obstacles denying them this ultimate self-determination.

It is argued that simply having access to lethal medications enables some patients to feel they have enough control over their fate to never use them. In the state of Oregon, many people die never having used the lethal medication that they have lawfully obtained there, under strict regulation. They are strengthened by knowing they can set their limits personally without depending on the unpredictable behavior of medical attendants who may, at the end, know very little about them.

No state makes suicide or attempted suicide a crime. Punishing those who assist a suicide may be the only circumstance in which there is a penalty for helping someone perform an act that itself is not illegal. Supporters of such laws argue that it is incumbent on society to discourage suicide, and, because it is absurd to have laws against suicide itself, punishing those who assist is the only way to evince a public policy of disapproval.

There are philosophers and physicians who say the profession would be ill advised to collaborate even "once removed" in a patient's self-administered death. However, there are also those who accept the enormous burden of doing their admittedly fallible best to evaluate the plight of each individual who asks for their help. They are aware that, in terms of outcome, refusing to participate is no less a decision than agreeing to participate. Although the primary purpose of a physician is to heal, when this is no longer possible, the next priority is to help, and to help in the way the patient wishes to be helped.

◡

With these ideas in mind, Roy and I talked it over.

My first response to Roy was a question. "I'm sure you've talked it over with her at length, haven't you? She's still on antidepressants, right?"

Roy assured me he had explored it thoroughly. He had made sure she had a "living will" and a directive refusing cardiopulmonary resuscitation (CPR). He told me he had even suggested a psychiatric consultation, but Norma had told him that of course she was depressed, and she couldn't see that a psychiatrist could change her situation. Wouldn't he be depressed if he couldn't do anything he liked and needed someone around most of the time to do just the simple daily maintenance tasks? Besides that, she was in constant pain and she could see no end to it. She knew that the prospects were that it would get worse, not better. "So," Roy concluded, "I think I'd do the same thing. It seems completely rational to me. Not only that," he added, "she's thought about it enough to have picked a date even before asking me. She wants to do it after the family get-together at Christmas. It would be over the weekend, when no help comes in for two days and Bobby, his wife, and the kids are visiting his wife's family."

"Did she speak to her son about it?"

"No, and she doesn't want me to, either, She told me she'd leave him a long letter and try to make sure he didn't feel guilty about it. She thinks he'd understand that nobody could make things better for her. They've gotten on well and..." He left the rest of his sentence unspoken.

We reviewed some of the literature about lethal dosage. Neither of us had reason to be knowledgeable about that. Roy decided that the method called "stockpiling" would be what he would speak to Norma about. Some medications are not lethal in small doses and could be prescribed on a monthly basis. If the patient collected them over a sufficient period of time, then took them all at once, they would cause rapid coma and death, usually within hours, often in less than an hour. There was time before Christmas to collect enough. I had not seen Norma for several years before Roy's call. I asked him to keep me posted on the events, and he promised he would let me know when anything happened.

⁓

Norma had awakened on a Saturday morning knowing she was going to be alone for the weekend. The cleaning lady had tidied up the house. Norma had asked for special thoroughness, and it was truly spotless. She had spent the morning putting together the papers she had been gathering for weeks. Her insurance forms, her funeral directions, all the bank account materials, and her will were piled on the kitchen table. She took care to lay out her "living will," hoping that in the event she had only partial success, no one would foolishly try to resuscitate her. She had looked over the family photo album and had gone through the contents of the box with ribbons and trophies and the scrapbook that documented her triumphs. She had decided she would have a nice lunch, already prepared, and then she would have her pills mixed into the pudding—she smiled at herself—"for dessert."

After assembling all the papers, including a long letter to Bobby with special messages for each of the grandchildren and a little tin box of chocolates for each of them, she decided she would shower. She undressed laboriously, using the special implements that assist arthritics in doing the tasks that healthy people take for granted. She caught a reflection of herself in the full-length bathroom mirror behind the door, and she stopped. She was always surprised at mirrors. They didn't replicate the young, vigorous, athletic woman whose image stubbornly persisted in her head until it was shattered by a mirror. It took a long time of painful self-delusion to rebuild this image until the next inadvertent encounter. The mirror showed a bent and elderly matron, stooped over, with gnarled fingers and toes, limping painfully despite hip and knee replacements, leaning on a cane that had been molded to fit her deformed hand. The hand itself had some dark spots around the fingernails where tissues had died from lack of a blood supply, and the fingers were twisted and distorted almost to the point of being useless. Only the special implements created for particular functions permitted her hands any utility. She saw the bent woman in the mirror enter the shower stall, sit on the special bench, and reach for the handle designed so that hands that could not grip a standard shower appliance could adjust it. She turned on the warm water and sat in the soothing stream; her tears mingled with the flow.

When she was finished, she reversed the tedious and painful process, using her tools to dress as well as possible, because she didn't want to appear disheveled to whomever chanced upon her. *I hope I don't alarm the cleaning lady*, she thought. *She's going to be the one who finds me, in all likelihood. Maybe I should leave a note on the table where she comes in and tell her to call 911 without looking in the bedroom. Yes, I think I will.*

When she had finished lunch and was ready for "dessert," she went into the bathroom again. She had hidden her cache of pills in their original containers—five of them that she had saved month by month, more than a lethal dose. She brought them into the alcove where she had eaten her lunch and sat down to prepare what she wryly called her "pudding and pill special."

↶

All together, I received three follow-up calls from Roy. The first was the Monday after the weekend that followed Christmas. He called me at home.

"Hi, Fred. Today I almost believed in ghosts."

That was an attention-getter. I had awaited his call about Norma with great anxiety and still some buried conflict about whether we had really done the right thing. "What? Is it about Norma?"

"Yes. She called me today, and I was shocked. I had expected a call, but not from her."

Remembering that her plan was to be carried out over the weekend just past, I asked, "Where did she call from?" Absurd scenarios flashed through my mind's eye.

"From home, of course, but I know what you're thinking. For a second, I thought I was crazy too."

"Well, what? What happened?"

"It's the most ironic thing you've ever heard. First, she told me she was calling long distance from heaven. I didn't know at first whether that was a joke or she had gone over the edge. Then she told me she had saved all her medicine for months, prepared everything in the house, and said all her goodbyes without revealing to anybody how permanent she believed them to be. She even had her helper buy her pudding to mix the medicine in so she could swallow it all."

"Okay, so what happened?"

"Believe it or not, she was laughing when she told me this over the phone."

"What?"

"Her arthritis is so bad she couldn't open the medicine bottles! She couldn't smash them and she doesn't have any tools, but she couldn't handle tools even if she had any. She just couldn't get to the medicine!"

If it weren't so serious, I thought, that sounded like the punch line from a sick joke. It took me a few seconds to gather my thoughts about all that had gone into that final outcome. All I could come up with was, "Wow! What now? What will she do?"

"That's what I asked her—whether she was going to try again. She said she's not sure when she can work herself up to that point again. She said if things continue the way they are, she will for sure. Anyway, she told me she asked different housekeepers and nurses to each open a different bottle for her. They have no idea she's even thinking about taking them all at once, but it's there for her now, if she wants. And you know? She still has a sense of humor. She told me she enjoyed the pudding."

It was only a few weeks after we celebrated the New Year that I received the second phone call about Norma. When I heard it was Roy on the phone, I thought I knew what he was going to tell me. I picked it up and asked, "Did she do it?"

"Nope. Now it's a real tragedy."

"Why? What happened?"

"Just exactly what she didn't want. Last weekend when she was alone, she fell off the toilet and hit her head. When she woke up, she couldn't get up, and she lay there 'til the cleaning lady came in on Monday morning. She said Norma was conscious but pretty incoherent. The cleaning lady called 911, and they rushed her off to the hospital. She was dehydrated, and she has a big ulcer on her side where she lay for maybe thirty-six hours. It looks infected. No cultures yet. They're not sure whether she had a stroke in the first place, but she's semicomatose. She's in and out of it. She can be roused and she answers questions some of the time, but it's not looking good. She's on IVs and antibiotics and vasopressors. Otherwise, her blood pressure drops off. They're at the point of deciding whether to start tube feeding."

"Her only family is Bobby, right?"

"Yes, but he doesn't know what to do. Will you talk with him with me? You know, she has a primary care doc, Latham, but she hasn't seen him very much because I've been managing the only real problem she has. Now, he's managing her because of the general problems, and I've never talked with him about the suicide idea. I don't know where he stands."

⌐

Roy was pointing up a problem patients encounter all the time.

Rarely have they spoken with their doctors about values and how they both feel about death and dying. What's more, there's no place a person may turn to find out in advance how any particular doctor feels about these important issues.

The Hippocratic Oath, which is often cited as if it could settle these difficult issues, deserves recognition for being an early public assertion of principles by a professional group. But persons who cite its authority usually select only the parts they prefer, leaving out, for example, the pledge of financial support for their teachers, swearing by pagan gods, and avoiding surgery.

The evidence[32] is convincing that admonitions against surgery, abortion, and euthanasia were the precepts of a small numerology cult, the Pythagoreans. Historical notice of the Oath was first made centuries after the death of Hippocrates. When Christianity became the dominant moral force in the Western world in that era, Christians found the Pythagorean oath compatible with their theology. They made use of it by appending Hippocrates' authoritative name, although what is prescribed was far from contemporary Greek and Roman medical practices. In fact, the ancient physician's direct participation in euthanasia (literally "a good death") by poisoning or phlebotomy was undertaken (along with the interdicted surgery and abortion) at the discretion of the physician upon the request of the patient. Further, from the actual Hippocratic corpus came the admonition to refrain from attempting to treat a patient "overmastered by disease." These things certainly don't support the idea that life must be preserved by all means and at any cost.

Of course, the fact that the Oath cannot be attributed to Hippocrates does not invalidate its precepts, just as its attribution to him is not an argument in favor of them. Quoting an ancient authority simply and arbitrarily cuts off discussion. It is better to discuss these issues in light of current knowledge and circumstances than to rely on slogans or authorities with whom not everyone agrees.

Today, codes of medical behavior that serve as guidelines have been developed by professional societies such as the American Medical Association, the American Society of Internal Medicine, The

American College of Obstetricians and Gynecologists, and the American Academy of Pediatrics. Basic ethical behavior of the physician is rarely part of the mandatory curriculum in medical school. The ethical precepts that guide physicians are more likely to have been gathered from examples at home or by life experiences as they matured. Some have had formal or informal religious or philosophical teaching. In other words, they have acquired their moral guidelines much the same way as non- physicians.

There are a great many ethical precepts with which most physicians agree, but there are no set rules to which a layperson may look in order to predict any physician's behavior in any given circumstance. Although a majority of the population, including physicians, identify themselves as belonging to a religious group, in a pluralistic society such as ours, there is no single authority for religious, moral, or medical truth.

A moral dilemma is characterized by a situation that demands a choice. It may be a choice between action and inaction or between two actions. But no matter which choice is made in a dilemma, some good will be done and some evil will be done, concomitantly. In confronting a moral dilemma, the task is to weigh and measure options in order to arrive at the better choice—the choice that will result in a proportionately better outcome. That is why ethics has aptly been called "the logic of tragedy."

⌒

Dr. Williams and I met with Dr. Latham at the hospital. We asked him what he thought about tube feeding. "We'll have to decide pretty soon," he said, "because she has not been taking enough food by mouth to sustain her. She only eats sometimes and then almost by reflex when we spoon food into her mouth. Her fluids are all IV. She's on pain meds, too, because the gangrenous areas and the huge back ulcer are really hurting her. She groans a lot, and dressing changes are bad."

"Do you think she ought to have a tube for feeding?" I asked.

"If it were me, I wouldn't want one," he replied.

"Have you talked to Bobby yet?" asked Roy.

"No, but he's coming over tonight."

"Did you know she wanted to commit suicide?" I addressed Dr. Latham.

"No, I didn't, but it doesn't surprise me. I guess that tells us how she'd answer if we asked her about artificial feeding. But she really doesn't have the capacity to give consent. She has a living will and a self-made do not resuscitate (DNR) order—you know, one of those CPR things. You signed it, didn't you, Roy?"

"Yes. Now we can meet with Bobby and explain why we don't recommend a tube. We're on the same page, right?"

"He doesn't know me at all," I said. "It's probably better if only you two spoke with him so he doesn't feel ganged-up on. I don't think you should mention the suicide idea. But maybe you can figure out how to tell him what Norma feels about going on with the pain and inability to manage her own life and do any of the things she enjoys. She may not survive infection and stroke anyway, and the vasculitis may already be affecting internal organs. Continuing all the supportive medications is really dragging out her misery. I hope he'll agree that she would refuse artificial feeding and blood pressure medication if she were awake enough. Call me, Roy."

⌐

Roy's third call about Norma came four days later. "She's gone," he said.

"That was very quick," I replied. "It certainly wasn't from lack of food and water. That takes two weeks. She was dying, wasn't she?"

"Yes, she had an overwhelming infection despite the antibiotics— we talked about stopping them but we didn't, we continued them— and her pressure just dropped out. The nurses and I talked to the family a lot. They all looked back fondly on the Christmas get-together and decided to remember Mom and Grandma that way."

"She certainly had miserable luck. Life's a tightrope, isn't it? You know what the worst thing was? It's really, really too bad she couldn't open those bottles."

PALLIATIVE TERMINAL
SEDATION

Despite the essential role that doctors have in caring for patients at the end of life, actions surrounding that critical time have become increasingly the province of the law, for the sake of public order and of religious beliefs. Laws serve to protect the vulnerable, which certainly includes the unwell. The story about Emma centers upon trying to help a patient achieve a peaceful death. It reflects a time before courts had, in light of new technology, reexamined the limits the law placed upon doctors attempting to achieve that goal. It was necessary to reevaluate the law because developing technology made it possible to prolong biological life long after biographical life had dissipated.

Some medical interventions appeared to me to be within the bounds of ethics and did not conflict with any established law. Based on a desire to benefit the terminal patient, and with some trepidation, I occasionally ventured into the gray space that the law had not yet ruled upon. Doctors, in their patients' best interests, took chances when they were treating patients near the end of life. We anticipated that, in time, the law would consider and affirm what we believed to be a humane medical rationale, necessarily respecting privacy and patient self-determination. That turned out to be true. The intervention I used with Emma is now called "terminal sedation." Emma's story about medical intercession at the end of her life started many years earlier, with her husband's illness.

~

By the time Emma could persuade her husband that spending money to consult a doctor for himself was not foolish self-indulgence, it was too late. Examination to evaluate what Mr. Klein called "a little heartburn," did not, as he expected, reveal the effects of dietary indiscretion but rather an insidious assassin lurking in the passage just above his stomach. Cancer of the esophagus had not only impeded the transit of his food, but its tentacles had spread to the surrounding tissues, invasive beyond the tools of medicine to overcome.

Hospice is a patient management concept for terminally ill patients. It changes the focus of intercession on behalf of patients from the curing to the caring elements of medicine. Concerned with the both psychological and physical elements, emphasis is on pain and symptom management and meeting emotional and spiritual needs. Supportive care may be offered in a live-in facility or in the patient's home. Hospice would have been ideal, but several years would pass before this enlightened concept was imported from England, first to Connecticut in 1974 and then early stirrings in Colorado in 1976. Unfortunately, there was no hospice in New York in the early 1970s, when Mrs. Klein sat helplessly witnessing the slow and painful dissolution of her husband. She had seen this robust man shrivel from 175 to 90 pounds, watching him become a whining parody of his aggressively independent and quite successful business persona. Pain relentlessly whittled away the strength and resilience that had enabled a once-penniless immigrant to forge a happy place for himself and his family in his adopted country.

When Emma could no longer physically manage her husband at home, she had sat by his bedside after he was hospitalized. At the recommendation of their family doctor, a specialist in a New York City hospital had taken over his care. The hospital where Mr. Klein was treated was one of the most respected medical school-affiliated hospitals in New York City, but, unfortunately, it practiced little of the palliative medicine—comfort care—that terminally suffering patients deserve.

Emma's timid requests to the nurse for more relief for her husband were met with, "That's all the doctor ordered," or, "I can't give him anything for another hour," or the very peak of irony, "More medicine might kill him." After her entreaties became punctuated with tears, the nurses took even longer to respond to the call bell. Emma suspected they found themselves unwillingly restrained, unable to exercise their judgment, and that they hesitated to face her or the patient with another protocol-bound refusal. She was beside herself with anguish from her helplessness in the face of authoritarian, seemingly callous, pronouncements. Couldn't they all see for themselves that he was dying, in terrible pain, and that they were offering no relief?

The residents and interns who visited did not stay long. They did not consider this a case where they could work a medical miracle— this was obviously a doomed man—so they moved on to someone for whom they had a therapy to offer. It was abundantly clear that no one had taught them how valuable a touch, a brief conversation, or some indication of empathy would have been to soothe the distress of the patient or his wife. They responded to Emma's plea for pain medication with useless advice—be patient and wait the interminable hours until the attending physician made rounds. When the attending physician finally did appear, he promised medication that was more effective. Perhaps the dosages were increased and maybe medications were changed, but Emma could detect no lessening of her husband's suffering.

Closer to the end, she found herself thinking the unthinkable. *I want him to die*, she thought. *How can it be that I want him to die? What horrible thoughts am I having? What is wrong with me? What kind of person am I that I want my husband, the father of my children, dead?* And when he did die, her grief was mixed with guilt, but guilt dominated her thoughts long after the grief had lessened.

ع

Almost ten years after her husband's miserable death, Emma Klein related this story to me at a Hemlock Society meeting (the group's original name after Derek Humphrey founded it in 1980). I had been asked to speak there about a new legal instrument for Colorado, called the "living will." It was designed to allow persons to write their wishes in advance of a crisis, in the event they became unable to communicate those wishes about end-of-life decisions when the time came. For most users, it served as a way to refuse "heroic" treatment, which, in their opinion, rather than prolonging life, merely prolonged their painful dying.

She was an ardent supporter of and recruiter for Hemlock, and she explained her motivation by relating the story of her husband's death. The objective of the Hemlock organization was to encourage legislation that would allow physicians to help terminally ill patients to die peacefully, if the patient decides that death is preferable to the suffering they are enduring. Emma hoped that such a law would be on the books should she be faced with a situation similar to her husband's. She wanted to avoid that tragedy and to enable anyone else of like mind to have means for a peaceful dying.

I explained to her that progress had been made in pain control over the years since her husband had died. What she was seeking, active euthanasia—which means a physician would administer a lethal drug to effect immediate death—remains illegal throughout the United States. Even if it were legal, I made clear, better pain management would make it a rare choice even for those who favor it. An alternative, physician-assisted suicide, is significantly different from active euthanasia. Medication, although prescribed by a doctor, is self-administered, thus it cannot be imposed on anyone. However, it too is illegal except in Oregon; in that state, a doctor, under strictly limited conditions, may prescribe a lethal dose of medication to be taken by mouth.

⁓

Several years passed before I saw Emma again. This time, it was as a patient. She reintroduced herself and refreshed my memory regarding our previous meeting at the Hemlock Society. She explained that her gynecologist had retired and she was in need of follow-up care. Three years before, she had had surgery and then chemotherapy for ovarian cancer. In fact, she had two operations. About a year after the first operation, after completing her chemotherapy, she had agreed to have her doctor take a second look. This was a frequent practice for an advanced cancer such as hers. She was greatly encouraged by the findings at the second operation, for there was no visible trace of the cancer. It had apparently been entirely removed.

I sent for her records and confirmed all that she had told me. She had had extensive surgery; even a part of the bowel had been removed where the cancer had invaded. For the moment, careful continued observation was the plan. I asked her if she had made an advance directive, perhaps a living will. Sheepishly she confessed she hadn't yet, but she had been meaning to, especially after her husband's experience and the findings of her first surgery. I asked if she had family nearby, and she explained she had moved to Denver after her second operation to be near her married daughter and grandchildren, although she lived by herself. Her son lived in Houston, and she had an older sister who had never married and still lived in the family home in Rhode Island. They corresponded occasionally but were not very close. Her sister, she told me, was very devout—more so than their now-deceased parents had been—and had considered Emma as the irresponsible younger sister whose frivolities had always been overlooked by their mother and, in particular, their father. Echoes of sibling rivalry resounded. Emma had the uneasy feeling that her sister had concluded, in some unfathomable way, that the death of Emma's husband and her affliction with ovarian cancer were somehow a reflection of her religious indifference.

Emma visited me annually, alternating every six months with her internist, who primarily managed her high blood pressure and mild adult-onset diabetes. It was with alarm that I received a phone call from him after her midyear visit with him. He told me she had complained of bone pain and that he had sent her for a scan. The report would be sent back to both of us. The report revealed metastases—colonies of cancer—that had spread to the bone. I called Emma, as I had agreed with her internist to do, and invited her in to talk things over; meanwhile, I arranged for a specialist in gynecologic cancer, a GYN oncologist, to manage the highly specialized care that would be the next line of defense.

We went over a living will together, and I recommended she speak with her daughter. She could, I reminded her, appoint her daughter to represent her wishes if she became unable to express them herself. Using the durable power of attorney for health care, she would have a legal advocate to represent her, especially to back up the wishes she expressed in her living will.

Over the next several months, Emma underwent x-ray treatment and some chemotherapy again, hoping the recurrent cancer would respond as the original one had. She did not visit me, because the treatment and side effects were managed well on an outpatient basis by the oncologist. For a few months, she appeared to be stabilizing, but she suddenly was stricken by a severe headache. Another cancer colony, in the brain, was diagnosed. I visited her in the hospital, and she, her daughter, the oncologist, and I had a conference. She was exhausted, drained from the irradiation and chemotherapy and aware that all her travail had been for naught. The bone pain, always just beneath the surface, began again slowly. The upshot was that she would transfer to hospice, where we would try to keep her comfortable.

After we left the room, her daughter called me aside and revealed that, although she had been appointed the agent for a durable power of attorney, she didn't think she could decline life supports for her mother.

Incredulous, I asked, "Even if she is being kept alive only so she will suffer more?"

"I just couldn't kill her." Eyes downcast, she almost whispered, as if the words were lethal. She looked up at me and repeated pleadingly, "I couldn't kill her."

"No, Lois, it's the cancer that's killing her. You have no control over that. But insisting on treatments like a ventilator or artificial feeding—that's only medical meddling. It only drags things out, prolongs pain and dying. People don't live forever, and cancer is what a lot of people die from, unless we interfere when we shouldn't. Anyway, it's against her wishes. She wrote that in her living will, and it's what she told you when she asked you to act as her agent for the power of attorney. She doesn't want any of those things."

"Well, maybe I shouldn't be her agent. I might ask for things to keep her alive. Maybe Donnie should. I don't know."

"Lois, you're here. Donnie's in Houston. Decisions may need to be made when Mom can't make them and we can't reach him right away."

"Oh, I don't know, I just don't know," she said desperately. "Maybe I won't have to."

Emma was transferred that evening. The oncologist had signed off from the management of her care because the metastases did not appear to be responding further to x-ray treatment or chemotherapy. I explained to Dr. Postin, the hospice doctor who took charge, that I had established a good relationship with the patient and would like to continue to consult on the palliative care that would be offered. The headache and bone pain were managed with strong medication, for a while. Emma seemed to be a little more cheerful having surrendered to the undeniable. Her children and grandchildren visited over the next few weeks, even those from Houston. But it was clear she was fading. She ate little and was visibly thinner.

The next blow fell almost simultaneously with the arrival of her sister from Rhode Island. The hospice doctor had learned the cramping Emma was having was not simply constipation from the morphine-derived drugs she was using; instead, the cancer was spreading, pressing on the bowel and causing a partial obstruction. I did not hear of this until after her sister phoned me indignantly, having learned on her visit to the hospice that her sister was on morphine for her pain.

"This is Stephanie Angel," she said. "I'm Emma's older sister, and what you're doing is euthanasia. Our family doesn't believe in euthanasia, and it's against the law. You tell them to stop the morphine immediately or I'm going to call the police!"

"Hold on a second, Ms. Angel. What do you mean, euthanasia? She's just getting medicine strong enough to control her headache and pains. Nobody's trying to kill her. We're just trying to make her comfortable."

"Don't try to pass that off on me. Morphine is what they use to kill people. I know that, and it's against the laws of God and man, so stop it immediately or I'll have you arrested."

"Well, I'm going to visit Emma after office hours today and I'll see what she wants. We'll go from there. Good-bye."

I went to see Emma and told her what her sister had said. She managed a feeble smile and said, "Stephanie is the least of my troubles now. Dr. Postin tells me I have a blocked bowel, partly anyway, and he's talking about surgery. What do you think?"

"I think we've got a lot to think about. Let's put it into the big picture, because that's where we are. You can't separate it from the rest of the cancer. First, the bowel. There are three choices: one kind of surgery, another kind of surgery, or no surgery."

"What do you mean?"

"Well, if we're going to relieve the obstruction before it blocks the bowel completely, we can try to take out the blocked part and hitch the bowel back so it works again as it did before. Of course, it can block again. Unhappily, that's not unlikely."

"What's the second surgery?"

"It's an easier operation and takes a lot less out of you, but the bowel doesn't work like before. It drains to a bag outside."

"You mean a colostomy?"

"That's right."

"Hey, Doc, that's a great choice you're giving me." She forced a wry grin. "What's the 'no surgery' choice?"

"Not doing any surgery at all."

Emma tilted her head. She looked directly at me and said, "You're trying to tell me that it's all over, right?"

I took her hand in both of mine. Meeting her eyes with mine, I said, "Right."

"Well, you said to look at the big picture. I've got recurrent cancer in my bones and my brain. About once every day for about a week now, I've felt as if someone is sticking an ice pick in my eye. It used to be for an instant, but now it lasts a few seconds. That seems to be getting longer. If that gets worse, I'm not going to be able to take it for long. So we're losing control over the pain, and now my bowel is closing down. Soon I won't be able to eat, even if I wanted to—which I don't, really. I haven't had any appetite for a week or so, and the truth is, I've only had a mouthful of Jell-O today. I'm just not hungry. I've had a pretty good last few weeks with the kids and all, except for the eye, right up to when the cramps started last Friday. And you know I don't want to go through what my husband did." She tugged on her sheet and pulled it up to her neck as if to ward off the inevitable. "What can I do?"

"Let me give you some generalities, Emma, and then we'll see what our choices are. One way or another, you're not going to be miserable like your husband was. We won't let that happen. But let me tell you what we used to do before we got a lot of high-tech stuff. People with cancer, stroke, or brain diseases like Alzheimer's would go to bed at home, friends would visit, and family would comfort them. And, just like you, most very sick people lose their appetite and gradually become undernourished and dehydrated. The family physician added opiates—that's the morphine family of drugs—to ease the passing and they'd die as peacefully as possible. So, let me ask you, are you uncomfortable when you eat so little?"

"No. I really don't miss eating. My mouth gets dry, but the nurse brings around some lemony swabs. Those right there." She puckered her mouth a little. "And I keep my lips moist. I sip a little water with my pills."

"Do you want to know why you're not uncomfortable now when you don't eat or drink much, or should we skip the explanations and just accept that's the way it is?"

"Yes, tell me what to expect," she asked, straining to sit up in bed and then leaning forward, still holding the blanket in front of her. "Mostly because I want to know if all of a sudden I'm going to wake up from a nap and feel starved and want to eat everything in sight."

"No, in fact, the less you eat the less you'll be interested in food. When the body runs out of sugar from food, it begins to break down muscle, and then nitrogen collects in the bloodstream. The marvelous thing about nitrogen is that it is a natural sedative. It makes you sleepy. That and the breakdown products from fat are nature's way of easing discomfort."

"Don't they put in feeding tubes when you won't eat?"

"I won't. Not if you don't want them. It wouldn't make sense for you. Keeping fluid balanced with tubes or IVs would simply prevent you from getting the sedative action of those chemicals your body is making."

"No," she pursed her lips tightly. "I don't want any tubes, but what about my blocked bowel and the cramps? And what about my eye?" she asked, squinting involuntarily.

"There will probably come a time when you'll have to choose between being awake with pain or being sedated so that you won't hurt anymore. We can make you unconscious, but that is a last resort. It will be your choice to make, if the time comes."

The time came all too quickly. Within two days, all the sources of pain had multiplied. Ms. Angel visited daily. I noticed Emma's increasing agitation after her sister visited, but unless Emma requested it, I had no authority to prevent visits. *Perhaps the visits are important*, I thought. This could be a time for reconciliation, as I'd seen often in families when a member was dying. I called Lois, who also visited daily and could see her mother's rapid decline. I told her the plan to increase pain medication and introduce sedatives that might soon make Emma unconscious. I suggested that Donald be called back from Houston for last good-byes as soon as possible.

Lois, Donald, and I had arranged to meet the next day, in the evening. When we met, I learned that Stephanie had also asked to meet them, but alone and before our conference. They had spoken at length and brought me up to date on the discussion they had completed minutes before.

They told me that Stephanie had started the conversation, "Thank you for meeting with me," she had said. "I know we've seen very little of each other as you've grown up, but you both moved away from home when you were very young, and I never could afford to travel. Your mother and I never saw eye to eye on most things, so I never got to know you. But this is very important for her sake."

Lois and Donald looked at her quizzically. What could this virtual stranger, who, as far as they knew, was alienated from their mother, have to say to them—as she had put it—for their mother's sake?

Stephanie continued, "You know what she and the doctors are planning, don't you?"

"Yes," Donald had replied. "Of course we do. The doctors told Lois, and Lois and I talked it over together. Lois is her agent for decisions."

"Did you know they plan euthanasia?"

"Don't be ridiculous, Stephanie," Donald had retorted. "She's dying of cancer. She's got it in her bones and her head and it's blocking her bowel."

"But they're filling her with morphine."

"Of course," Lois had said. "She's in terrible pain."

Stephanie looked at the ceiling and then back and forth between Lois and Donald. "Don't you see? She never came to the Lord. This is her chance to be with the Lord in his suffering. They're interfering with that. They're blocking her feeling. This is the chance He's giving her before she dies. Before they starve her to death."

Lois had responded, startled, "Starve her to death? No one said anything about starving her to death. I told the doctor I'd have trouble stopping life support." Turning to Donald, she asked, "Feeding is life support, isn't it?"

"Yes," Stephanie interjected. "Of course it is. They can't do that."

Donald raised both palms out in front of his chest in a universal gesture. "Hold on a minute. We've got a conference scheduled with the doctor in about fifteen minutes. You come too, Stephanie. Let's get all the questions answered. Lois, you seemed pretty sure about what was happening on the phone."

"Well, I was. And Mom was sure."

I was a little surprised to see Stephanie there with Lois and Donald, since she had been so hostile to me and had avoided meeting me at Emma's bedside each time I had visited before. Nevertheless, after hearing their conversation reiterated, I decided I'd start at the very beginning and explain the plan. I was aware that their mother was perfectly capable of making her own decisions and that Lois, as her agent, had no say in the matter while Emma was still capable. Yet their grief was apparent, and everyone would be well served if they understood the plan and were in agreement as death approached.

I began with the same sort of thing I had said to Emma. "Technology and modern medicine have great things to offer, but if they're used unwisely, they add to misery. Your mother," turning to Stephanie, "and your sister, is terminal. I would not think she could survive as much as two weeks more, probably days. She is having increasing pain, and like most seriously ill people, she has no desire to eat."

Stephanie interrupted, "But you could put in a feeding tube. You don't want her to starve to death." Turning to Lois, who was crying silently, she said, "You're not going to let her starve, are you?"

I turned to Lois, who had shrunken into herself and buried her face in her hands as Stephanie threw the last accusation at her. "Please hear me out, Lois. Then I will answer any questions you may have, but let me tell you, the word *starvation* has no place here." I went on, "When someone loses her appetite and stops eating and drinking, she begins to use up her own tissues for energy. That's why anyone would lose weight after the sugar reserves are gone. Muscle break-down causes nitrogen to build up in the blood. It acts as a sedative, and fat breakdown causes a condition known as ketoacidosis. That's the substance that causes diabetics to slip into a coma. Both of those things would be a relief for Emma."

Directing my next comment to Stephanie, I continued, "It's bad for a diabetic with nothing else wrong, but for a dying patient, it's a providential way of easing the passing. It's the natural way as it was meant to be before well-intended but ill-advised artificial hydration and nutrition came along. In this case, technology serves only to allow patients to be awake and aware of their discomforts, as opposed to peacefully slipping away. You're wrong if you consider a dehydrated and undernourished moribund patient who has no appetite to feel the same way as you would if you skipped breakfast, had no time for lunch, and got home very, very late for dinner. You would be greatly misinterpreting the circumstances. I don't think—and what I think or don't think doesn't matter, so let me start over. More important, Emma doesn't think that prolonging her dying now makes any sense. Everything we're doing is to help with the pain and make her dying peaceful."

"Then you're going to knock her out." Lois seemed relieved. She dried her eyes and her face relaxed.

"If that's the only way I can keep her from the misery she's in. She's the one who asked me to hold off—but only until Donald could get here. She told me to ask you not to bring the children, because she's so miserable that she can't disguise it. If it had been up to me, for her sake, I would have sedated her yesterday. But she's calling the shots."

༄

What we were planning in the early eighties for Emma became progressively more widely practiced for terminal care. It was given the name "terminal sedation." In the context of advanced disease and expected death, terminal sedation refers to a last-resort clinical response to physical suffering that cannot be relieved any other way. Rendering the patient unconscious is to relieve suffering, not to end life. *Terminal* doesn't indicate that the purpose is to terminate life. The right to refuse artificial nutrition and hydration was upheld in the 1990 Cruzan case.[33] The U.S. Supreme Court ruled that a person may refuse any medical treatment, even life-saving treatment. Even later, in 1997, when the U.S. Supreme Court ruled[34] that there was no constitutional right to assisted suicide, Justice O'Connor addressed the use of pain medication for the terminally ill: "in these states a patient who is suffering from a terminal illness and who is experiencing great pain has no legal barriers to obtaining medication, from qualified physicians to alleviate the suffering, even to the point of causing unconsciousness and hastening death."

Briefs to the Supreme Court from hospice and geriatric groups that opposed physician-assisted suicide stated that terminal sedation and cessation of eating and drinking were morally and clinically preferable last-resort alternatives because the physician does not directly or intentionally hasten death. Both sedation and refusal to eat and drink can be undertaken and supported within usual health care settings.

Contrast this with assisted suicide, in which the patient dies from an extrinsic factor—namely, the lethal medication that a doctor must prescribe—not from something related to the illness. Many clinicians who oppose physician-assisted suicide, yet do not want to abandon their patient, find that the option of terminal sedation provides a morally acceptable way to respond to severe terminal suffering without violating their conscience.

Justice O'Connor was utilizing the "principle of double effect." Intention is the significant factor when "double effect" is cited. When one performs a good or neutral act, an evil outcome may be foreseen, but it is not intended. Giving pain medication to a suffering patient is a good act, but it may result in a foreseeable but unintended shortening of life. The intention is pain relief, not curtailing life. The outcome is proportionately good. Therefore, the act is morally acceptable.

~

When I had finished, all three members of the family appeared to understand. Donald and Lois accepted that relief of her suffering was the most important value for their mother. I'm not sure that was Stephanie's first priority, but in the face of Emma's clear wishes and the acceptance by her son and daughter, she capitulated and made no further protests—at least to me.

We all went to Emma's room. She put on a bold front for her children, but her furrowed forehead reflected the constant pain, and her facial features tightened spasmodically, reflecting intermittent paroxysms. I explained to Emma that we had all spoken about the plan she and I had made. I asked her when she wanted me to start the intravenous medications that would make her pain-free. I reiterated that, once the medication was started, it would gradually make her unconscious within an hour.

Lois, who had been sitting at the bedside, asked Emma, "Is it okay if I come onto the bed?" Emma put her arm out and around her as Lois hitched herself up and laid her head on the pillow beside her mother. Donald pulled his chair up close and held Emma's other hand.

Emma said, "Good. I want to talk privately for a while with Donald and Lois. Then I want to start the medication." Turning to her children, she said, "I'm sorry to have such a short time to say good-bye, but you can see, the pain is getting to be unbearable. Stephanie, please understand. I really appreciate your coming to see me and your truly good intentions. We haven't been close for many years, but underneath you're my sister. We shared a lot when we were children, and I've always loved you. I hope you understand."

I imagined how, many, many years before, Lois might have climbed into her mother's bed and been comforted, as she was being comforted now. Her trembling chin was surmounted by a paradoxically beatific smile, belied by silent tears. The tips of the fingers of Donald's hand that Emma was squeezing were white, and the pressure spoke volumes to him, reassuring him more than words that the right choices were being made to ease his mother's last hours.

I excused myself after assuring Emma that I would return in an hour, or sooner if she wished, to begin the protocol that would make her pain-free. I ordered an IV with both sedatives and opioids to be ready. When I returned in an hour, Stephanie was gone. I felt sorry for her and hoped her ego hadn't been damaged significantly by the rebuff, however apologetically it was worded. My main concern was for Emma and her children. I also felt confident that Stephanie's faith was strong enough to sustain her.

We started the IV. Emma drifted off to sleep with Lois and Donald beside her. I explained to them that when dehydration and malnutrition alone cause death, it takes twelve to sixteen days. I did not think this was going to be the case with their mother. Emma, as we had planned, never awakened. Her course was not protracted, and she died on the third day after starting the sedation, clearly from her cancer. Her children took some solace in that.

CHOOSING

In the late 1980s, ethical quandaries about end-of-life treatment were being examined closely because of the impact of technology. It was a time of transition, a time when doctors were wrestling with legal and ethical uncertainties concerned with the discontinuation of life support. An artificial breathing machine, the ventilator (also called a respirator), had been employed in the past as a "bridge" to sustain life for short periods of time while damaged organs healed or toxins were metabolized.

There had been a precedent for extended use of life support. Before the Salk vaccine virtually eliminated polio beginning in 1955, an earlier type of respirator had been employed, the "iron lung." It was a long and wide airtight metal cylinder invented in 1928, used primarily over the next three decades for polio victims. Patients who couldn't breathe because the virus had paralyzed their respiratory muscles were sealed inside with only the head protruding. By alternately raising and lowering the air pressure within the large cylinder, the patient's chest would be compressed and expanded, and air would be forced in and out of the lungs, like a bellows. Today, this device has been almost completely replaced by the ventilator, a much more compact breathing machine that is attached to a tube entering the patient's windpipe.

I don't recall any debates at that time about whether to use the iron lung for a paralyzed patient. In the days of "doctor knows best," whenever a treatment was available, it was used. Neither can I find reports in the media or medical literature of that era about patients asking that it be stopped to permit them to die. It was not until many years later that the "right to die" became an issue for heated public debate. The media portrayed the patients confined to iron lungs as heroes, survivors through extreme adversity. They were not accused of using resources that could better be diverted to lives that were more productive. In that era, there was neither publicly funded Medicare nor Medicaid, nor talk of rationing. Death was accepted as an outcome because "everything had been done." In those days, "everything" was a lot less.

⌁

Many years had passed since the era of the iron lung, and I was about to be called upon to help a family and their doctor with the dilemma of discontinuing life support. I had just come home from the office for dinner, and there was my phone message machine, blinking its red eye at me. I listened to a call from one of the newer family physicians on staff. She had left her home number, asking if I would call after seven that evening. She had a problem regarding care of a patient, and an older partner in her group had suggested she contact me.

After dinner, I went into my study and called her. "Hi, Dr. Abrams," she said. "Thank you for returning my call. I'm sorry to bother you at home, but Dr. Lindstrom suggested I speak with you because you have a special interest in medical ethics. He told me you helped get the Colorado advance directive law passed, so I thought you might have some ideas that might help—about the law, I mean, or if you've heard about a situation like this."

I asked her to tell me her patient's story, just as we all had learned to do in medical school. What was the "chief complaint"—that is, the immediate problem—and then, what led up to it. Apparently, she had difficulty trying to phrase the immediate problem, having not had to deal with it before for a patient for whom she was responsible. It was too complicated, she explained, for her to compress it into a simple "chief complaint." For me to understand, she needed to start with the background first.

She reported that her patient, a Mr. Schwartz, had amyotrophic lateral sclerosis, and she'd been caring for him since she began practice in Denver a year and a half ago. During her narrative, I became aware that Dr. Baron was speaking in short bursts, rapidly and breathlessly. She was clearly distressed as she described the inexorable paralysis that was consuming her patient, ascending from his lower body to his chest. Breathing problems are inevitable in persons as they progress to the later stages of ALS. The ironic thought flittered through my mind that, in her agitated speech, she was reflecting her patient's agonizing inability to breathe.

More than a year ago, she had discussed with Mr. and Ms. Schwartz the relentless nature of the disease, explaining measures that could be taken to ameliorate the symptoms as much as possible, but nothing that would change the ultimate outcome. She had told them that he would soon need artificial assistance to breathe, a ventilator. It would force air into his lungs through a tube attached to a metal device surgically inserted into his trachea, through a tracheostomy. Putting it in under anesthesia would not be painful and, once it was there, it wouldn't hurt. But several times a day, a suction tube would need to be inserted into his windpipe to clear the secretions from his lungs.

More than a year had passed, but, as predicted, the time came that he could not breathe without assistance by a ventilator. Dr. Baron told me that before she scheduled the tracheostomy, she had reviewed with Mr. and Mrs. Schwartz the additional difficulties that would be encountered. There would be new communication problems because the tracheostomy prevented speech. Words could be mouthed silently, but breath was short-circuited before it could pass through the vocal cords. The incision site needed special hygiene, she told them, to avoid infection, and she reminded them that additional secretions could be expected in the windpipe that would have to be suctioned out.

By this time, Mr. Schwartz was confined to a specially purchased hospital bed. He required twenty-four-hour nursing for all the functions we take for granted—basically, he had to be fed and helped with bowel and bladder evacuation. He needed to be massaged, bathed, and turned to relieve pressure on his skin. Good round-the-clock nursing care kept Mr. Schwartz free from infection and skin ulcers.

During these difficult times, their rabbi visited the Schwartzes frequently. Their religious beliefs were of great solace to them, but they had not yet completely addressed with their rabbi what guidance their religion offered as Mr. Schwartz's life options slowly diminished.

Jewish beliefs and practices vary widely among the three basic branches—Orthodox, Conservative, and Reform. All, however, have a presumption toward preserving life. Overwhelming suffering is considered worse than death, but that never justifies suicide or murder. Just as for many other religions, life is considered a stewardship, on loan from God, and not to be disposed of autonomously. Suffering is not invited, but it is possible sometimes to find meaning in it. The Orthodox depend primarily upon strict rabbinical interpretation of written law that directs that everything possible must be done to prolong life. The Reform are less legalistic, tending toward a covenantal relationship with God. Individuals are empowered to make moral decisions based on their personal conclusions, but they are expected always to respect religious teachings and to seek counseling from a rabbi.

To help the Schwartzes consider their options, the rabbi related words of guidance from a compendium of civil and religious rules that supplement the Old Testament. This compendium, called the Talmud, is composed primarily of rabbinical legislation and commentary recorded during the first through the sixth centuries. Of course, in these early writings, there could be no literal precedents for the techniques and knowledge of modern medicine, so contemporary decisions are based on rabbinical interpretations made over many centuries, from studies of ancient histories.

Their rabbi recounted to them a centuries-old description of the last days of a venerated rabbi who was in overwhelming distress, both physical and emotional, as he was dying. His disciples prayed fervently for his recovery. His maidservant believed these prayers were cruelly prolonging his dying—merely postponing his inevitable death and protracting his agony. She smashed a clay vessel on the floor, and the noise so startled the disciples that they stopped their prayers for just a moment. But this brief lapse allowed the rabbi to slip peacefully away.

"Many scholarly commentators," the rabbi explained, "find support in this story for removing obstacles to death when it is inevitable." As we have learned to expect, in most of the tales related in historical holy writings there is invariably a contrary narrative to ponder and weigh against the first. "From the Talmud and over many centuries thereafter," the rabbi continued, "respected rabbis have reiterated other teachings that militate against hastening death in any way, considering the shortening of life—even by a moment—tantamount to murder. There are specific prohibitions against several actions, proscribed because they were believed to hasten death, such as moving a dying person, or closing his eyes or removing his pillow. Even preparing a coffin in advance of death has been condemned."

The sum of the conversation with the rabbi made it apparent that there was no certain, clear direction to be derived from the teachings. Was a ventilator in this case prolonging dying or preserving life? This narrow area was left to the patient to weigh and balance. Refusing or accepting life support was something for each patient to decide. Because of the strong traditional presumption to always choose life, without prompting by the rabbi, Mr. Schwarz and his wife, Anna, resolved that if assisted breathing was necessary for him to stay alive, then that's what they would do.

Speaking with the tracheostomy in place was not possible. Fortunately, the patient had used a computer in his daily work before he was stricken with ALS, so he was already using a keyboard and screen to communicate. They made up macros so he could press a single key to indicate he was hungry, or to say "thank you," "that's enough," "I need a blanket," and other simple phrases. As it progressed, the paralysis left him with little more than the ability to swing his arm with a finger pointed to hit the keyboard.

At the time of this episode, for a patient to be at home with professional, round-the-clock nursing care and a ventilator was a new venture, still bordering on experimental. Today, it remains a difficult and expensive, if less rare, option. It is not feasible in every home environment. Mr. Schwartz's life was completely dependent on total body maintenance. Even breathing was mechanical, with an electrically-driven breathing machine backed up by a generator in case of power failure. If that too should fail, there was a last-resort manually operated bag-and-mask.

Dr. Baron, it appeared to me, had offered everything she could in keeping with the goals of Mr. and Mrs. Schwartz. When she completed the story, explaining the situation right up to her house call today, I prompted her with, "Yes, and…?"

"That's the problem; he doesn't want to do it anymore."

"Do what?"

"He wants to quit the ventilator."

"Yes?"

"Well, wouldn't that be committing suicide—and if I discontinued the ventilator, wouldn't that be assisting a suicide?"

By then, courts had established legal presumptions for considering end-of-life decisions. One presumption was that action should be taken to prevent suicide. The important point, I told Dr. Baron, is that a presumption is only a starting point. Argument and evidence can reverse it, just like for another familiar legal presumption, "you are innocent until proven guilty." I recalled a decision by a wise judge who had carefully examined the presumption regarding the prevention of suicide. The patient under consideration, like Mr. Schwartz, was suffering from ALS and did not wish to live the rest of his life on a ventilator. The attorney general in Florida had threatened to indict anyone for assisting a suicide, a felony under Florida law, if they helped the patient to discontinue the ventilator. The judge, in his thoughtful decision affirming patient self-determination, pointed out an essential fact: the patient had not inflicted ALS on himself. The inevitable death was the natural course of the disease and could not possibly be considered as suicide. The ventilator could be refused by the patient and removed without fear of prosecution of his caregivers.[35] Although this issue was settled in Florida, the U.S. Supreme Court had not yet affirmed a constitutional right to refuse medical treatment. That was established twelve years later in the Cruzan case.[36] Reasons for starting a respirator and circumstances when it could ethically be discontinued were still uncertain; law, ethics, and religion all had their say. Subsequent experience, common practice, and, in some cases, court decisions have clarified many dilemmas since then; nevertheless, decisions about life and death are still hotly debated despite law and practice precedents.

"But once I started the ventilator," Dr. Baron interjected, "wouldn't it be like me killing him if I took it away?"

"How do you feel about that," I asked. "How you feel is pretty important."

"I—I don't know," she mulled.

"Well, let's go back to the time you proposed the ventilator. Suppose he had refused. Would you have forcibly anesthetized him to do a trach and then would you have tied his hands down so he couldn't pull it out when he woke up?"

"Of course not. First of all, I'd need consent to do an operation, and, anyway, I wouldn't treat a patient who doesn't want it."

"Right," I said. "So what's really going on here? Are you taking away a respirator from Mr. Schwartz, or is he simply refusing a treatment?"

"But it's started," she protested weakly.

"Sure, but when he went on the ventilator it was something he'd never experienced. Most people grab for anything that will prolong life. It's only when the quality of their life is so badly diminished that they realize they'd prefer death. You'll see more of this when you get to take care of more patients who have symptoms that move beyond our ability to control, like shortness of breath when their lungs are damaged, or pain so severe that it can only be managed by making them unconscious. Lots of unconscious patients are placed on ventilators after a stroke or a head injury. You don't know then if they'll ever be able to breathe on their own again. If they do, that's been a successful trial of treatment. If they don't recover, nothing has been lost. You may find out after a while that they won't recover from an injury, or they might not want to continue postponing death by using an artificial breathing machine. They might feel they're just prolonging dying. And both the doctor and the patient have learned something you didn't know when you started. So wouldn't it be foolish to persist in a mistake just because you started one? I mean, you couldn't know then if it was going to work until you tried."

"Of course, that's true." She began to think aloud. "Otherwise, if we thought they barely had a chance, we'd skip a lot of trials—especially if we had to continue it forever even when we found out it was wrong. Then the rare patient who might recover wouldn't have been given any chance at all. But for Mr. Schwartz, now we know. There's no question. He's not going to get better. He's really refusing treatment, isn't he? It's different when you know the prognosis." She continued, summing up her conclusions. "And it's not hard to sympathize with someone in his predicament. I don't think I'd do anything different for myself. But you've got to be there to make the decisions. I mean, he's got to decide. Nobody else could do that." She invited me into her train of thought, asking, "What do I do now?"

"Well, have you spoken to his wife? Was she there when he asked you? What did you say to him? What about the rest of his family?"

"Yes, he used his computer, and it took hours to write a long message to his wife about it before he wrote to me. In fact, what he did was show me the message he'd sent his wife with a short message to me explaining."

"What did he say?"

"Well, the essence of it was there was nothing left in life for him except thinking about his death, which was imminent. So he wanted to go out with what little control there was left to him."

"And you told him...?"

"I'd get back to him tomorrow."

"What did his wife say?"

"She believes it's his right to decide, but she had two other concerns. What would their children say about it, and what would their rabbi think."

"Well, we certainly have to speak with her ASAP, and the rabbi, too. Can we get together tomorrow?"

"I'm sure we can. The rabbi has been very accommodating, and Anna—sure, she'll want to meet."

"Let's set up a meeting at noon tomorrow. After that, we'll all need to get together again and include their children."

"And we should include the psychologist who's been working with them since he came home from the hospital the first time with the ventilator—and the nurses who've become so attached to him and the family."

We met at Dr. Baron's office at noon the next day. Dr. Baron explained what Mr. Schwartz wanted to do. The rabbi turned to Anna and asked, "Did you know this?"

"Yes."

"What do you think?"

There were no sobs, but tears slowly trickled down her cheeks as she spoke, looking down at her hands in her lap. "I don't know what to think. It's been terrible for him—for all of us. And we don't talk any-more—I mean with the computer. He just lies there. It's terrible. He should do what he wants, but the children—" She dabbed at the tears and turned to the rabbi. "What is right—what are we allowed to do?"

"Allowed? You remember the Talmud. Are we prolonging dying? If that's what's happening, we don't have to do that. We shouldn't do that. Impediments to a peaceful death may be removed. He may refuse treatment that merely prolongs dying."

Anna appeared to be greatly relieved. She addressed no one in particular as she ruminated, "And the children?" Their children were mature young people, both in colleges nearby. The boy was nineteen and the girl twenty-one.

We discussed the plan to have a meeting with the children and all concerned as soon as we could. I would explain the plan, and Dr. Baron would add details as called upon. But first, we agreed to visit Mr. Schwartz that evening, as Dr. Baron had promised, to make certain of his wishes and to review with him and the rabbi any remaining doubts about the acceptability of withdrawing the respirator. Before we left, after we had set up the evening meeting, the rabbi asked, "How exactly do you do this?"

I answered because Dr. Baron had no experience to cite. "When we're sure that's what he's determined to do and we're satisfied that he's able to think clearly, then we ask him if he has decided when to discontinue the respirator. Then we explain that we'll give him a sedative that will allow him to sleep and, when he's asleep, we'll turn off the respirator."

"Oh, wait!" the rabbi said. "We can't do that."

"What? What is it we can't do?" I asked, softly, not challenging but rather asking for information.

"Isn't making him unconscious—I mean, if you give him morphine or whatever it is you give him—isn't giving him medicine causing his death?"

"No," I explained. "Being unable to breathe is causing his death. He's refusing the respirator, and we're not going to force it on him. We're not going to demand that he pull it out by himself and then stand around while he's gasping. Death will come in a few hours, maybe less. It depends; he may be able to breathe a little on his own. But we're going to do what we do for any patient in distress: give medication to relieve it. It's the paralysis of respiration—from the ALS—not medication, that he's dying from."

"Of course," the rabbi murmured, looking across the room at nothing that was visible to me. Then more audibly, he explained, "I just hadn't thought about the actual—actions. I've just heard people talk about 'pulling the plug,' and that was that. I hadn't thought about it. I mean, I hadn't pictured exactly what happens—the sequence of things, I mean." He turned to me. "But really, there's nothing else, nothing else you could do—of course, but keep him comfortable." And, almost as an aside to himself, "Whatever it takes."

We met with Mr. Schwartz that evening. Communication was difficult, and we framed our questions so they could be answered by nods or shakes of the head or the yes-no buttons on the computer. Ultimately, we all were satisfied that he had made a competent decision. He had chosen a date. We explained the process and agreed to meet with his children and the other caregivers in three days, enough time for the children to come home for the meeting.

We met early in the afternoon three days later. Anna had called the children, Sandra and Samuel, and told them that there was going to be a meeting with all the people who were taking care of their father and it was important that they attend. They assured her they would be there, and both had arrived that morning. Everyone was prompt, and we settled down in the living room, where Mr. Schwartz lay in his special bed with the computer at his fingertip. We introduced ourselves, although the family knew the nurses and the rabbi. I introduced myself last as a physician and a consultant "on situations such as your dad finds himself in now." Momentarily, I turned my head toward the nurses; then I faced the children, who sat together on a small sofa. "You all know what your dad is going through and how bravely he has faced his illness—and mom, too. The respirator has assisted him to breathe for more than a year now, but as every day passed, he lost more of his physical abilities. Now, he can do nothing for himself. He has told us he feels trapped in a body over which he has no control, and he doesn't want to live this way any longer."

Both children, the nurses, Anna, and Dr. Baron were crying silently as I recounted the unremitting events. I turned to Mr. Schwartz and asked him if what I had said correctly expressed his feelings. He nodded and pressed his keyboard to record a "yes" on the screen.

"What does that mean?" His son's voice was shrill with alarm. "What do you mean?"

"He has asked us to turn off the respirator," I replied, and then I could no longer suppress my silent tears. "He won't be able to survive without it, and he knows that. Is that right, Mr. Schwartz?"

Again, a nod and a computer signal, "yes."

"When—when will you do this?" his daughter asked.

"Wait, wait" his son interjected. "I don't want to know."

I addressed Mr. Schwartz: "You've picked a time?" He nodded.

Anna spoke. "He's told me. He hopes everyone will be here. I will tell Sandra and the rabbi when. Dr. Baron will be here, of course, and the nurse or all the nurses may be here. If Samuel doesn't want to be here, that's all right." She turned to Mr. Schwartz. "It's all right, isn't it? We'll call him after."

Samuel sobbed, "I'll be back in a minute," and fled the room. Sandra embraced her mother; they both turned to Mr. Schwartz. Anna looked into her husband's eyes and reached for his hand as Sandra grasped her father's other hand. The rabbi said he would like to ask for a blessing, and we stood and bowed our heads as he prayed in Hebrew. I didn't understand what he said, but I felt a blessing was truly merited for those who, while drowning in grief, sorrowfully responded to the entreaty of a dying man—a brave man pleading only that he be understood for asking that an impediment to a peaceful death be withdrawn.

THE OLD MAN'S FRIEND

Ah! I thought. *A good Monday morning. Only one new admission overnight.* I had begun rounds early in the hospital that morning, not knowing what to expect. As usual, I stopped at the nurse's station and pulled the one new medical record from the roster of admissions that my associate had left for me after his night on call. There was the chart of a Mrs. Odin, admitted to the medical unit with a diagnosis of double pneumonia.

Unusual, I mused. *She was sick enough to admit to the hospital but not bad enough for the intensive care unit* (ICU). Then I spotted her age. She was seventy-four. Something was awry. Usually, an older person with severe pneumonia will be undergoing vigorous treatment, most often in the ICU. My concern changed to astonishment when I turned to her order sheet. There were orders for diet (whatever she wanted), ambulation with help, oxygen, small doses of morphine for "discomfort," and something for sleep. But where were the blood counts, and the vital signs of pulse, temperature, and blood pressure? And most alarming, what antibiotic was she on? None appeared on the order sheet. Mrs. Odin was critically ill with a diagnosis of double pneumonia, a disease that was readily treatable—but no one seemed to be doing anything about it!

The sudden realization that a serious error had been made sent an electric jolt into my chest. I turned to the nurses and asked who was caring for Mrs. Odin. Shifts had just changed, and I had missed the nurse who had admitted her. The current nurse had no more information to offer, having just come on duty, and she knew only what had been reported to her by the departing nurse—namely, that my partner, Dr. Cartwright, had left orders for management. I read the brief admission note that he had scribbled in the just-after-midnight hours. He wrote that Mrs. Odin was a long-time patient whom he knew well. The diagnosis was pneumonia affecting both lungs. The medical history and physical examination had been dictated,(but not yet transcribed), he wrote, and he would leave appropriate orders. I decided I had better phone my partner before I visited the patient.

I caught him at home just coming out of the shower, getting ready to go to the office to start the day after a night on call.

"Hey! What's up with Mrs. Odin?"

"Oh, sorry, I should have left you a little more info. Sorry, but I thought her daughter would be there. Did you see her?"

"No, I thought I'd better speak with you first because you didn't leave any real orders for antibiotics and—"

"Sure, I left orders, but her daughter didn't want any antibiotics."

I was tempted to say with just a touch of sarcasm, "Then don't give her daughter any, just make sure the patient gets them," but I didn't voice my first thought, because I didn't want to sound flippant about such a serious matter. Anxiously, I told him I didn't understand what was going on. Why wasn't he treating an elderly woman with pneumonia with antibiotics?

He explained that her daughter, who was her caregiver, had brought the patient to the emergency room. The ER doctor had called Dr. Cartwright at home because he was confused. The daughter, Mrs. Rind, a mature woman, had explained that the patient had Alzheimer's disease and that she, the daughter, was her agent with a durable power of attorney. Her mother had begun coughing two days earlier, and it had gotten worse—bad enough to take her temperature, which proved to be quite elevated. At about this time, her mother, Mrs. Odin, began having significant difficulty catching her breath, and that's when Mrs. Rind brought her to the ER.

The ER doc listened to her chest and ordered an x-ray, which demonstrated pneumonia affecting both lungs. He had explained to her daughter that he wanted to admit the patient to the intensive care unit for oxygen and antibiotics. At that point, Mrs. Rind had said she wouldn't give consent for antibiotics. The ER doctor, after a difficult night on duty, was a little testy.

"Then why did you bring her to the hospital?" he asked.

"Because," Mrs. Rind quickly replied, "she is uncomfortable with the cough and can't catch her breath."

The bottom line was that the patient herself appeared to be confused, agitated, and uncooperative. She had refused antibiotics with a perseverance that almost seemed scripted. But if there were doubt about her ability to make competent decisions for herself, then her daughter, as her agent with a durable power of attorney, was empowered to make medical decisions on her behalf. She, too, had emphatically refused antibiotics for her mother.

This rather complicated situation needed extensive evaluation, and a busy ER was not the place to undertake it. Knowing that Dr. Cartwright was her primary physician, rather than become embroiled in a debate at that late hour with her daughter over proper care for pneumonia, the ER doctor called him and asked him to come over and manage the problem.

⌐

Indeed, it was confusing and complicated, with a long story behind it—a story dealing with an issue that a wise physician had addressed a century before Mrs. Odin was born. "Pneumonia is the old man's friend," Sir William Osler had asserted. This highly respected physician was referring to nature's way of sparing a patient a protracted, painful demise at the end of a long life. Over the intervening century, even the definition of "old man" has changed. At the beginning of the twentieth century when Osler made his comment, Americans could expect to live forty-seven years. Now, in the United States, both men and women can anticipate surpassing the biblical three score and ten by more than seven years

Of course, we have all encountered people of advanced years who are enjoying good health and mental alertness, while others of less-advanced age are scourged by ill health and mental incapacity. Rather than asserting glib generalities about how many years a life should last, we've learned that how a person functions is more important than chronological age. We must always raise the question, "Shouldn't we ask the 'old' man (or woman) if (and when) pneumonia may be a friend?"

↵

As the story unfolded, I learned that Mrs. Odin had been a respected and well-loved high school English teacher. After mandatory retirement, she had refused to let her experience and talent go to waste, so she volunteered to teach the English language to recent immigrants. She had an ear for language and soon found herself learning Spanish while she taught English, so she no longer had the handicap of "one-way" communication with her students. She found her new task even more rewarding than teaching in high school, because these students, usually older and more mature than those in her high school classes, were happy to be there and eager to learn. An avid reader, she introduced English literature to some of the more-advanced students, and together they enjoyed reading and translating short stories by John Cheever, Eudora Welty, and Ernest Hemingway.

Neither mother nor daughter had paid much attention to what they both believed were the annoying but laughable incidents that occurred intermittently over the next few years—Mrs. Odin was forgetting names, misplacing objects, wondering why she found herself in front of the refrigerator, and, after a moment, remembering. But rather suddenly, Mrs. Odin's husband, a lifelong smoker, began to have trouble with a racking cough. Within three months, he was dead of metastatic lung cancer. This loss appeared to affect Mrs. Odin profoundly in many ways, but disorientation was the most obvious.

After her husband's death, she had returned to teaching classes, feeling it would help her adjust to the loss of her husband and companion of more than forty years. Ordinarily, misplacing car keys and eyeglasses are such common failings that they are the subjects of much wry humor among older persons. As the months of mourning continued, however, Mrs. Rind began to observe that her mother was having difficulty beyond everyday forgetfulness. She began to spend more time with her mother, who confessed that she also had noticed her problems were increasing significantly. She couldn't always remember her students' names in class, and she was frequently distressed when she could no longer quote favorite passages from her beloved stories, novels, and plays.

Unhappily, Mrs. Odin decided she had to give up teaching. At that time, her daughter urged her to move into her home, where there was enough space for her to have a large bedroom with an alcove she could use as a sitting room; this setup allowed her to have privacy and a retreat, when she wished, from her daughter's children and husband. Reluctantly, she gave up the independence that came with having her own apartment.

Mrs. Odin did not wish to be a nuisance by becoming dependent on her daughter, who had her own home and her children and husband to deal with, as well as her own social life to live. She was aware that to become isolated was an invitation to mental stagnation. She decided to drive to the new senior center, where activities were planned around the needs of retirees who wished to remain active. Perhaps, she thought, she might find new friends, maybe even a book group of contemporaries.

Instead of leading her to a haven, the expedition proved to be a terrible turning point. She found herself unable to identify the streets once she left her immediate neighborhood, despite the fact that they were merely extensions of those streets with which she was familiar. She felt her heart begin to beat faster as she searched for a place to turn around and return home. Suddenly, she faced an oncoming truck and she became shockingly aware she was going the wrong way on a one-way street. Frantically, she swerved into a driveway as the truck driver shouted something and drove by. She could barely catch her breath, and perspiration spread on her scalp as it had when she was going through menopause. Mrs. Odin sat stunned for a moment and tried to catch her breath.

A sympathetic young woman appeared from the house whose driveway she had entered, responding to the blaring horn and screeching tires.

"Are you all right?" she inquired through the half-opened window.

"Yes, yes, I—I think so."

"Can I help you? Would you like to come in?"

"Oh, no, no."

"Are you lost? Can I call someone for you?"

Mrs. Odin became calmer, regained her composure, and rationally asked if she could use the phone. She called her daughter, who drove the short distance to her location and, after assuring herself that her mother was once more in control of her senses and her car, drove slowly, leading her home.

The experience was so unnerving, however, that Mrs. Odin surrendered her driver's license. She began to have intermittent episodes of uncharacteristic grumpiness, especially with her grandchildren—with whom she had previously been very indulgent. In fact, her daughter had complained she was "spoiling the kids." She began to have difficulty balancing her checkbook, unusual for a woman who had managed the household expenses and even dabbled in stock market investments. At this point, it was no longer possible for Mrs. Odin and her daughter to deny that a problem existed.

Mrs. Rind consulted with Dr. Cartwright about her mother's symptoms, and the doctor advised her that it sounded much like Alzheimer's. Testing would be important to try to rule out other causes of dementia, some of which were amenable to treatment. They discussed how to break the idea to Mrs. Odin, because many persons with Alzheimer's are in denial, he explained, and they become quite defensive at the suggestion they are not thinking clearly.

"Some patients in an early stage," he expanded, "when they understand their condition and the dreadful prognosis that comes with it, become badly depressed. The depression virtually paralyzes them, and that cheats them out of the few years left when they still might enjoy some of the pleasures of life. We used to avoid telling them their diagnosis because of that. But," he continued, "there is much more emphasis on self-determination these days, and less tolerance for just blindly following 'doctor's orders.' People don't want doctors simply telling them what to do anymore. So, if your mother is still able to function well mentally, I think we should give her the opportunity to discuss the future. That leaves her with some control, even though we—and she, too, of course—all have to face what we know is going to happen. We probably still have a short window of time to let her know about it while she's well enough to understand. We'd be denying her that chance if we delay much longer."

Mrs. Rind, well aware of her mother's native intellect and the spirit of self-reliance, which had so recently been assaulted by many small failures, agreed that she would not play the role of mother to her mother. With some trepidation but a deep-felt conviction that this was the proper way to show respect, she acknowledged that informing her mother fully was the better choice.

"Besides," she told Dr. Cartwright, "thinking we could wait until she loses it all and doesn't know enough to care—no, Mother's too smart for us to pretend nothing's wrong. We've already talked about it some. She won't buy it—that nothing's wrong, I mean."

Very shortly thereafter, Dr Cartwright had a lengthy visit with Mrs. Odin, whom he had not met before. He focused especially on her mental agility, using various simple tests of memory, her ability to calculate, and the like. He asked her about her activities—what she did around the house and for entertainment. He told her the possibilities, the many different reasons for occasional confusion and memory loss. He asked about her diet, probing for a vitamin B-12 deficiency and about medications and alcohol consumption, but she ate intelligently, drank only an occasional glass of wine, and was taking only vitamins and calcium—nothing that could affect her thinking. After the physical exam, he asked her to return when test results were back to discuss the findings.

While she was waiting for her next visit, Mrs. Odin further demonstrated her initiative and intelligence by going to the Internet. She was quite familiar with searches because the World Wide Web had previously been a source of great pleasure for her when she explored the literary sites. This time, the information she collected was far from entertaining.

When she returned to the doctor's office, she brought with her much material gleaned from the Web—including the widely used staging information detailing the inexorable progression of Alzheimer's disease, which ended, without respite, in death. After the tests, including the Mini Mental State Examination, were completed, the doctor came to the inescapable conclusion that she had early Alzheimer's disease. But he was pleased to be able to demonstrate that she still retained the capacity for making critical decisions.

Mrs. Rind had accompanied Mrs. Odin on that visit. She was aware of her mother's research but was unwilling to discuss it until Dr. Cartwright had established the diagnosis. She needed time to get used to it, but she was pleased that her mother took the initiative in gathering more information, unlike many less strong-willed persons, who, in the face of illness, sometimes allow themselves to be infantilized.

"Let's talk turkey, Dr. Cartwright," Mrs. Odin began. "You suspect Alzheimer's and that's what you've been testing me for, isn't it? After the material I've read, I think that's what it's going to be. If it's Alzheimer's, is this pretty much what's going to happen—the stages I've read about, I mean? Here they are."

She handed him the pages she had taken off the Internet.

She went on, "This list that's written and the order of—I guess deterioration is what I'd call it—has been around for a long time, but the disease doesn't seem to have changed. Has anyone come up with treatment since then?"

"First," said Dr. Cartwright, "you're right about what I was looking for, and you figured it out for yourself. It looks like Alzheimer's. You know that's a diagnosis we make from all the signs and symptoms and some tests, but mostly it's by eliminating the other possibilities."

"But you can be pretty darn sure, can't you?" she asked. "I read that the only absolutely certain way to diagnose it is a brain biopsy, and I suspect there are not a lot of volunteers for that."

"You're right there, and I don't know any doctors who ever were willing to chase the diagnosis that far either," Dr. Cartwright added.

"And there's not much to do about it, right? I mean, it's going to happen, isn't it?"

"Well, there are some new medications they're trying. They're on the market, and some people say they slow the process down."

"They slow it down? Okay, but do they stop it?"

"No," he said as he put his hand on her arm."

"So, you're telling me that, if I live long enough, I'm not going to recognize my friends, my daughter, or my grandchildren; I'm not going to be able to read or figure out the television schedule or use the computer. If what this says about progressive deterioration is true, I'll be a baby again. Someone is going to have to change my diapers?"

Dr. Cartwright nodded.

"You know," she said matter-of-factly, "I don't want to live like that."

She paused for a moment and then asked, "How long does this take, before I'm completely gone? I don't mean mentally; I mean how long do I live this way?"

Doctor Cartwright replied, "I can only give you statistics about that. That depends on how bad the symptoms are when it's diagnosed—and women live longer than men, too. And whether or not any other illness comes along."

"Okay, so what are you saying?"

"Well, you're seventy now, and looking back, you've had gradually increasing symptoms for about three years, right? You're a teacher, so you know about statistics and what they hide. The median survival for someone your age is about eight years, but the range is as much as twenty. You really don't have any other health problems, like diabetes or heart disease, that shorten life even more."

"Isn't that great," she responded in a voice heavy with sarcasm. "Now I can live a nice long time just falling apart."

Because there's nothing good to say at such a time, Dr.

Cartwright offered, "We'll always be here to care for you. I know your daughter and her feelings for you, and she'd never abandon you or let you suffer."

"No, that's not the point. I've always treasured my books, poetry, the beauty in a not-so-beautiful world. I can't let that person—me—turn into a shabby, nasty, incoherent, smelly old lady that's a burden to anyone she comes into contact with. I must think about this."

They left, making another appointment for a week later to discuss options for care and treatment. When they returned, Mrs. Odin had made some decisions and had talked seriously and deeply with her daughter. The first thing she asked was about suicide. Would the doctor provide her with medication that she could take if the situation became unbearable?

Dr. Cartwright did not answer directly.

"Mrs. Odin, the operative words in what you're asking me for are, 'if the situation became unbearable.' The problem with that idea is that otherwise healthy persons with Alzheimer's are not necessarily very sick—you won't necessarily have significant physical symptoms until way late in the illness. By that time if, as you say, things become unbearable, you wouldn't have the mental ability to plan or voluntarily take medications. You wouldn't even know—I mean you wouldn't be your same self any longer. But later, you'd have symptoms; you'd feel discomfort. You'd just be too disoriented to do anything about it. You wouldn't think coherently. Patients at that stage can't even figure out whether their clothes match, let alone plan a suicide. Their caretakers have to help with pain or distress. And, of course, that's what I and the family would be doing, making sure you're okay."

"Well, what can I do?" she pleaded.

"The best thing to do is to write down how you want to be treated under the circumstances that might arise as these stages progress, and then appoint someone to represent you to make sure everyone does what you want. But remember, no one can give you deadly medicine. It's against the law even if you found a doctor willing to do it."

"I could stop eating, couldn't I? They couldn't stuff a tube down me if I didn't want it."

"You're right, no one can force any treatment on you that you don't want, and feeding tubes are treatment that you can refuse like any other. But it's hard to quit eating. If you didn't do it right away, while you're thinking about it and made up your mind that's what you are determined to do, the ability to think clearly goes away and you would probably forget what you wanted to do. By that time, somebody would have to feed you and, whichever 'self' you are, you'd probably accept spoon-feeding. It's sort of instinctive. You probably couldn't form a true intention to refuse, and no one would deny you a bowl and spoon. More than that, they'd feel obligated to offer it to you, as long as you were conscious and not refusing, although they probably wouldn't force a tube on you. Unfortunately, the symptoms you want to avoid, like loss of control of bowels and bladder, unexplained aggression, the dementia—these come before the appetite goes. It's different from illnesses where the body goes before the mind does. The fact is, legally, you can refuse any treatment at all, but you must make your wishes clear. Write them down and figure out who you would want to make decisions when you can't any longer. I would guess that would be your daughter. Is she your only child?"

"Yes, and she'd be the best to ask, now that my husband's gone."

Dr. Cartwright referred her to the local Alzheimer's support group, where they helped her fill out a combined living will and durable power of attorney for health care. She spelled out her wishes, making it clear that she wanted no treatment for anything that would prolong her life, no matter what illness befell her. Any medical intervention should be directed only to making her comfortable. If a choice ever had to be made between comfort and shortening life, comfort was her choice. Clearly, during follow-up visits and talks, they had determined that neither Mrs. Odin, Mrs. Rind, nor Dr. Cartwright was a "vitalist" who believed life must be prolonged for its own sake. For them, quality of life trumped sanctity of life beyond doubt.

Mrs. Odin appreciated that her disease was a fatal disease, and, worse yet, one in which the longer you live the more severe the symptoms. Unless it was essential to keeping her comfortable, it made no sense to treat an intercurrent disease during the course of Alzheimer's in order to prolong her life. That would simply increase the probability of deterioration to a worse stage with more discomforts. Mrs. Odin did not choose to stop eating, because there was still time for enjoying ice cream, and windows of lucidity for understanding books and poetry. She reiterated at every opportunity that it would be good if there were an easier way to die. Sometimes, she wryly asked Dr. Cartwright if he had any nice, quick diseases she could catch.

It appears that four years after the diagnosis was made, Mrs. Odin got her wish, a providential illness that could ease her way. And there I was, on rounds. I understood my partner's wisdom in discreetly complying with the patient's choice. Neither Dr. Cartwright nor I believe that it is a doctor's duty to use all the tools in the black bag to prolong life.

The orders Dr. Cartwright left were designed for Mrs. Odin's comfort. Hospital routines were cancelled—no repeated blood tests, temperatures, breath counts, and blood pressures, that would disrupt her rest without adding relief.

On rounds, in the clear light of morning, there were several things I did not do. It has been my experience that hospital protocols are established for the safety and welfare of patients with the patient's best interests at heart. Under some circumstances, however, their routine interventions become unnecessarily intrusive, especially to a critically ill patient. I did not call in the risk management department, because they would have been obliged to investigate a deviation from "standard" treatment. The patient and her daughter would have had the distress of defending to strangers their very personal decision, which clearly had been an anguishing resolution, made only after careful weighing and balancing. Of course, the patient was in no condition to participate at all. Dr. Cartwright assured me he had seen the papers, they were in order, and they soon would be on the record.

There have been cases in which a person, often unrelated to the patient, has a deep religious conviction that life must be prolonged whatever the circumstances. Unsolicited, they have involved the legal system, which then became obliged to investigate. This does not add peace to a dying patient's final days.

Our past experience with the ethics committee convinced us that they would have strongly endorsed the management plan we had chosen, which was compliance with her refusal of anything more than treatment for symptoms. Nevertheless, contacting the ethics committee would have called for another meeting and further intrusion. I didn't call them.

I called the social worker and explained the situation. I knew there would be need for grief counseling for Mrs. Rind and the grandchildren, when they visited. I spoke with the nursing staff and explained why the patient was in an ordinary room, not in ICU, and why her treatment was for symptoms only. I told the charge nurse that either Dr. Cartwright or I would be glad to speak with any staff members if they felt the patient wasn't receiving proper treatment. Indeed, in this exceptional situation, the pneumonia treatment was secondary to the patient treatment that was appropriate, treatment for relief of the existential suffering of which the patient had written in her advance directive and spoken of to her daughter and Doctor Cartwright.—the knowledge of the ultimate progressive deterioration of Alzheimer victims. Perhaps a meeting regarding Alzheimer's care and management could be scheduled if she felt one would be helpful.

Pneumonia spared Mrs. Odin the implacable, inevitable progress to the later stages of Alzheimer's disease. The children did not suffer the bewilderment of not being recognized by their grandmother. The family did not experience the exhausting loss of communication and the exasperating repetition of questions with the same answer. She did not suffer confusion while she was trying to comprehend who the strangers were that intruded upon her living quarters and shared her food. She and the family did not have to cope with the disruptive and anguishing confrontations that paranoia brings, such as accusations of theft should she have misplaced her belongings. All were spared delusional and violent behavior that might have developed, perhaps resulting in painful injury to her or her caregivers. Such occurrences would have been incomprehensible to those who knew her as a gentle person.

They did not have to make the agonizing choice of sending a beloved family member off to be cared for by strangers, to be isolated or perhaps put in restraints for her safety and the safety of others. This fastidious woman did not survive long enough to deteriorate to the point where she would need diapering for urinary and fecal incontinence, or bathing by a caretaker, a necessity many Alzheimer's patients misunderstand and fear. She did not descend to the ultimate indignity for a literary devotee—end-stage mental incapacity with a vocabulary depleted of all but a half-dozen words; she wouldn't find herself unable to smile, sit erect, or hold her head up. Indeed, for Mrs. Odin, not for a moment did we doubt that pneumonia was the old man's—and woman's—friend.

CONFESSION WITH
TONGUE IN CHEEK

There's no way to deny it—I deceived my neurology professor. I can no longer confess to him—he is long gone to his heavenly reward—so I must confess to you. Let me assure you, no one was harmed in any way, so I have forgiven myself on his behalf. In fact, I look back upon it as a stroke of good fortune that I earned. I earned it because, like my fellow students at Cornell Medical College, I studied and studied, and when I was finished, I studied some more. Studying makes no physical demands, yet we were still exhausted at the end of the day. One of the students raised this issue with the professor one day, in a class on calories and metabolism. The student speculated that the calorie consumption must be enormous for continuous studying. He hopefully suggested that despite midnight snacking, he wouldn't gain weight. This balloon of wishful thinking was quickly deflated. Half a handful of peanuts, the professor informed us, could more than sustain the brain work of a week of studying.

But I digress. I have to go back more than half a century to explain about my deception. All of us had eagerly awaited what we students called "the clinical years." At that time in the history of medical education, the first two years of school were devoted largely to the basic sciences—anatomy, physiology, biochemistry, and the like. Time dragged by because it seemed we were not progressing beyond an exponentially more intense undergraduate premed curriculum of basic sciences. We were all anxious to get into real doctoring—taking care of people and making them better. We used to make fun of each other with the grandiose statement that we had better hurry to get out there and "save lives and relieve suffering." But we really meant it!

Each of us was thrilled to don a white coat, secure a stethoscope, and have our own ophthalmoscope for eye exams, and a little black bag with a kit for making blood counts and urinalysis. We were clinical clerks who trailed after interns and residents, duplicating their efforts by taking another medical history and doing another physical exam. We often became closer to the patients than the house staff could because we saw fewer patients and we spent much more time with each individual than the "real doctors." We returned from our sallies into the New York Hospital, Payne Whitney Psychiatric Hospital, and Bellevue and exchanged tales of our experiences. I remember one of my classmates, whom I shall call Peter Swanson, because that wasn't his name. Peter was a blond, blue-eyed, apple-cheeked young man who always looked freshly scrubbed—even cherubic. That's probably what got him into trouble. His assignment was to take a history from an inpatient in the psychiatric ward. He appeared in our post-excursion huddle with a bruised eye, which we suspected would soon be a "shiner." He explained he had entered the room of a frail, elderly, white-haired lady who was lying in bed reading a book. He could see it was embossed in gold on the cover, *Holy Bible*. As he entered, she looked up, smiling, and said, "How nice—you've come to visit me."

"Yes, Mrs. Thompson. I would like to ask you some questions, if I may."

"You are so kind," she said, "and pure and beautiful. Come closer."

"Thank you," Peter replied as he approached the bed. "May I sit down?" he asked, moving to the chair at the bedside.

As he arrived next to her bed she crooned, "Yes, like an angel; you look like an angel."

Peter didn't quite know how to respond to this effusive greeting, so he just sat down.

Mrs. Thompson continued, "In fact, you look like Jesus." And with that comment, she drew back her hand holding the Bible and slammed it into Peter's face, shouting, "Now, Goddammit, turn the other cheek!"

As I recall, that was the only physical assault any of us suffered during our clinical years, although none of us emerged without a bruised ego from merciless quizzing. Interns and residents badgered us with progressively more complex questions, stopping only when we got to a detail that we couldn't answer. Then they told us to go look it up.

My most ignominious moment came on the obstetric service. This future obstetrician/gynecologist had never witnessed a birth. Few twenty-four-year-olds with an urban upbringing had. I was thrilled that I was going to be permitted into the delivery room to see a baby actually being born, as long as I stood well off from the action. I donned my scrubs, mask, hat, and shoe covers, and slid against the wall far behind the obstetrician. The patient was very noisy, and I had never seen or heard anyone in such continuous distress before. It was unnerving, and I wondered why they were not alleviating her pain; just at that point, a gush of bloody fluid splashed far and wide as the baby slithered out. In fact, there was very little actual blood loss, but the red-tinged amniotic fluid appeared to me to be gallons of blood, and I was certain the patient had exsanguinated before my eyes. Happily, the new mother had stopped crying out and began cooing. I also realized the floor and walls of the room had become very unsteady, so I quickly left the room and gulped the air in the passage outside, where I also found a chair. For a very few minutes, I wondered if I should have gone to law school.

I might add that I did not think for a moment about the invasion of privacy my presence denoted. I had been invited to observe and I went, eager to learn. In retrospect, I doubt anyone asked the patient, an indigent woman who was being cared for at no charge, for consent to permit entry to an observer who played no role in patient care. In the 1950s, informed consent was still a novel process in medical care.

I suppose that is why I didn't notice that male students were egregiously uninformed when they agreed to be sperm donors. This is another ethical problem that I look back upon fifty years later. This time, I was the "victim." As resident doctors or medical students in the fifties, we were called upon to be sperm donors. We thought of it only as a ridiculously easy way to make ten bucks. That really made us vendors, not donors, but the terminology has stuck. The donation technique was introduced as a medical process in 1884, but its successful use was not revealed for another twenty-five years—when a young man who had been born as a result of the process revealed it to an astonished world. When this first case of the use of artificial insemination was made public in the early 1900s, it was denounced as mechanical rape, adultery, and against the laws of God.

By the time we students were asked to participate, two generations later, sperm donation and artificial insemination was a standard procedure, though secret and anonymous. Genetics was in its infancy, and the only testing was a medical history casually asking for any known familial disease. I doubt I would be wrong in saying that none of us thought we ought have any responsibility toward the new life that we might help create. We didn't give it a thought! None of our mentors, the respected attending OB/GYNS who asked medical students for sperm, ever raised any issue beyond our being on time and entering through the back door of the office. No one suggested there was anything to think about! Admittedly, we were adults, but to say the least, adults woefully unsophisticated. Our education was sorely lacking in philosophy. We had been much too busy seeking the grades that would get us into medical school. We had not been cautioned to consider the significance of our actions. Our "consent" was woefully uninformed.

⁓

Those were our adventures "uptown" at my "home base" at 68th Street and York Avenue. But Bellevue Hospital was a different world. It was the hospital of last resort in New York City. Cornell University Medical College, New York University Medical College, and

Columbia University Medical College shared the responsibility for indigent patient care there. It would be more than a decade before Medicare and Medicaid were established to offer care that was other than charity. We students were responsible for doing the simple laboratory work on all admissions. We did blood counts to detect infection or diseases such as leukemia. We did urinalysis to detect acute or chronic kidney diseases. It was a great responsibility, as it was a first screening for serious illness. When we had to draw larger quantities of blood, we needed to take a sterilized syringe and needle from the antiseptic soak they were in. There were no disposables then. Everything was sterilized and reused, including the rubber gloves for examinations or surgery. The length of rubber tubing used for tourniquets for drawing blood from the arm had a way of disappearing, so we simply had a fellow student place two fingers just inside the short-sleeved gown and twist until the sleeve squeezed the arm enough to make the veins stand up. We called that maneuver a "Bellevue tourniquet." Because drawing blood is a two-handed procedure, if no colleague was available, we had the patient slide the fingers of his opposite hand where ours would have been; holding the sleeve tightly until we drew the blood.

This is what I remember of events fifty years ago. It may have become distorted by time. The emergency room at Bellevue bore a disturbing similarity to Grand Central Station. The main floor was a long rectangle that looked like a basketball court. It may have been one at some time. The periphery was divided by movable screens perpendicular to the walls, making booths about ten feet square with a gurney cart in each. Scores of patients were being sorted—we called it triage. Around the entire wall, fifteen or twenty feet up, was a balcony. The attending doctors and advanced residents stood there with megaphones, directing the actions of doctors and nurses on the floor below as patients were shunted in and out, to and from various destinations.

That's the venerable institution where, I must confess, the deception occurred. After lecturers had presented the didactic material on various subjects to us, part of our final exam was to examine a patient, report what we believed to be the diagnosis, and explain the basis of our conclusions. In a teaching institution, part of the challenge and learning opportunity among the faculty and young doctors was a continuous intellectual game of stump your colleague—or better yet, harass a student into being constantly on the lookout for the esoteric and bizarre. Painful as it was to us students to be reminded of our relative ignorance, that approach continued to increase our powers of observation. It also had some less helpful results. We had fewer exposures to the commonplace, the things that practitioners see daily. For example, I saw three cases of leprosy before I ever saw anyone with measles. The older teachers were beyond that game, pointing out that students should first look for the obvious. They had an adage: "If an animal is galloping down Main Street, it's probably a horse and not a zebra." Nevertheless, at examination time they often would spring traps. Perhaps they concluded that if we could dissertate on the rare, they could assume we knew the commonplace.

It was with trepidation that I traveled to Bellevue to take my oral exams in physical diagnosis. I was not sure I was going to be able to identify the undoubtedly exotic disease that the instructor had selected to challenge my diagnostic acumen. We were not allowed to look at the chart or laboratory work. The diagnosis was to be made based on a physical exam and the patient interview.

My first clue to a possible diagnosis was the fact that they sent me to the neurology section. *Uh-oh*, I thought. I didn't feel too sharp in neurology, and I began to worry more. I approached the bedside of a woman in her thirties and introduced myself. "Good afternoon, Miss Stover. I am a medical student, and I understand they have told you that I was coming to speak with you and examine you as part of my training."

"Yes, they ask me to come in several times a year for exams. I think it's more for your exam than mine." She smiled and I smiled in return.

"That's probably true, although I'm sure it's good for you to have regular checkups. Anyway, it's very kind of you to come in so we may learn to help other people with their illnesses. I appreciate your willingness to help me become a good doctor." I didn't think it would hurt to be friendly rather than appear like an aloof professional doing her a favor by being there. In fact, I thought, it *was* nice of her to do this.

"Well, you're much more polite than the last student I had. He just poked and prodded me as if I were a turkey he was considering for Thanksgiving. I'm sure he flunked."

We both smiled again, but mine was more like a nervous grimace. I replied, "You've got a very colorful way of describing things, Miss Stover."

During our conversation, I had noticed that her speech was slightly slurred and her lips were forming each word with an effort that showed speech was difficult. It was forced, like some people I had encountered with cerebral palsy. I saw that her skin had a slight yellow tinge. I had no clue as to what this all meant. I asked if I might look more closely at the whites of her eyes. I pulled a chair up close to the bed.

"Oh," she said, "you noticed that, too—the yellow. I have jaundice."

"Yes. Is that the symptom that made you come to the hospital?"

"Well, the first thing I noticed was I was becoming clumsy with things. I sew a lot, and I was dropping things."

"Anything else?"

"Yes, when I reached for thread or material, my hands began to shake."

"That must be awful for someone who uses her hands for fine work," I said sympathetically. "Did you make that beautiful shawl you're wearing?"

"Yes, and that embroidered bag with my comb and lipstick and stuff."

"Well, they're very elegant. Do you sell them?"

"Oh, no. I just make them for myself and for friends." She coughed slightly as if she needed to clear her throat.

"Let me get you a glass of water," I said as I rose from the bedside chair and reached for the pitcher and glass.

As I handed her the water, I saw her hand movement change from a smooth reaching motion to a shaky tremor as she came closer to the glass. A little of it spilled, and she said, "See what I mean?"

"Yes. That must be very frustrating for you."

She replied, "You're very sympathetic." Then she smiled coyly, tipping her head to the side, and asked, "Are you married?"

Startled, I replied, "Yes, very happily, very happily."

"Oh, well, you're too young for me anyway. But—since you're so nice, I'm going to tell you what I have. It's Wilson's disease. It's a genetic disease of copper metabolism. Most people get it at a younger age than I did. The liver becomes overloaded with copper and it goes all over the body."

I was taking notes frantically.

She continued, "The clumsiness is due to dystonia secondary to brain involvement. Are you getting all this? I can slow down."

"No, you're—that is, *I'm* doing fine. Go on."

"What brought me to the hospital was what they called an 'oculogyric crisis.' My eyes rolled up into my head, and I couldn't move them for maybe ten or fifteen minutes. I drooled and my tongue stuck out. That scared me, so I couldn't ignore things any longer. Then I came here and they did some tests. I don't know what it is, but my ceruloplasmin was low. But you know what gave it away for certain?"

"No," I replied, eagerly awaiting more pearls of wisdom to flow from those eloquent if rigid lips, which were guiding me to an A in physical diagnosis.

"I have Kayser-Fleischer rings!" she announced.

I looked at both of her hands and could see no adornment. "Kayser-Fleischer rings!" I exclaimed. "Where are they?"

"Come closer and look in my eyes," she said.

I feared we were getting back to the marriage thing, so I said, "What do you mean?"

"My eyes! Around the pupil. Look!"

I looked closely and saw distinct rings circumscribing the pupils of both eyes. They were greenish gold in color and very striking. I searched the furthermost cranny of my mind for even the slightest recollection of any reference to a ring-around-the-iris and eureka! It dawned on me that it was copper deposited from the faulty metabolism of which she had spoken, deposited there, as it was throughout the body, because the liver, unable to dispose of it, "overflowed."

As the cliché goes, "The rest is history." I stunned the professor with my astute observations, which were missed by many of my seniors on first exam. I even spoke about the mysterious ceruloplasmin to help clinch the diagnosis, along with the now (for me) golden, rather than simply copper, Kayser-Fleischer rings. It was wonderful!

Many years ago, Sir William Osler, a much respected and widely quoted role model for physicians, advised his students, "Listen to the patient...he is telling you his diagnosis."

Never did I expect this aphorism to be translated so literally—I got an A.

BIBLIOGRAPHY

Annas, George J., *Standard Of Care,* Oxford University Press, New York City, New York (1993)

www.avert.org "The History of AIDS" 1987-1992, 1993-1997, 1998-2002, 2003 onward- last update 8/2005

Battin, M. Pabst, *Ethical Issues In Suicide,* Prentice-Hall Inc., Englewood Cliffs New Jersey (1982)

Beachamp, Tom L., Childress, James F., *Principles Of Biomedical Ethics 5th Ed.,* Oxford University Press, New York City, New York (2001)

Beers, M.H., Berkow R., eds. *The Merck Manual,* Merck Research Laboratories, Whitehouse Station, New Jersey (1999)

Black, David *The Plague Years* Simon And Schuster, New York City, New York (1985)

Blackburn, Simon, *Being Good,* Oxford University Press, New York City, New York (2001)

Bok, Sissela, *Lying,* Pantheon Books, New York City, New York (1978)

Byock, Ira, *Dying Well,* Riverhead Books, New York City, New York (1997)

Callahan, Sidney, Callahan, Daniel eds., *Abortion,* Plenum Press, New York City, New York (1984)

Cameron, Peg ed., *The Physician and the Hopelessly Ill Patient,* Society For The Right To Die, New York City, New York (1985)

Copeland, Larry J. ed., *Textbook Of Gynecology 2nd ed.,* W. B. Saunders Company, Philadelphia, Pennsylvania (2000)

Domurat Dreger, Alice, *Intersex in the Age of Ethics*, University Publishing Group, Inc., Hagerstown, Maryland (1999).

Engelhardt, H. Tristram Jr., *The Foundation Of Bioethics*, Oxford University Press, New York City, New York (1996)

Faden,Ruth R., Beauchamp, Tom L., *A History And Theory Of Informed Consent*, Oxford University Press, New York City, New York (1986)

Graber, Glenn C., Beasley, Alfred D., Eaddy, John A., *Ethical Analysis of Clinical Medicine*, Urban And Schwarzenberg, Baltimore, Maryland (1985)

Humphry, Derek, *Final Exit*, Dell Publishing, New York City, New York (1991)

Jaffe, Carolyn, Carol H. Ehrlich, *All Kinds Of Love*, Baywood Publishing Company, Inc., New York City, New York (1997)

Jonsen, Albert R. *The Birth Of Bioethics*, Oxford University Press, New York City, New York (1998)

Jonsen, Albert, Siegler, Mark, Winslade, William, *Clinical Ethics 5th Ed.* McGraw-Hill Companies, New York City, New York (2002)

Lattanzi-Licht, Marcia, Mahoney, John J., Miller, Galen W., *The Hospice Choice*, Fireside, New York City, New York, (1998)

Lewis, C.S., *The Abolition Of Man*, MacMillan, New York City, New York (1972)

Monagle, John F., Thomasma, David C., *Medical Ethics* Aspen Publishers, Inc. Rockville, Maryland (1988)

Monitoring Stem Cell Research: A Report Of The President's Council On Bioethics (Pre-Publication Version) Washington D.C. (2004)

Morowitz, Harold J., Trefil, James S., *The Facts Of Life* (Oxford University Press, New York City, New York (1992)

Pellegrino, Edmund D. Thomasma, David, *For The Patient's Good* Oxford University Press, New York City, New York (1988)

Reich, Warren Thomas ed., *Encyclopedia Of Bioethics,* Simon & Schuster MacMillan, NewYork City, New York (1995)

Robertson, John A., *Children Of Choice,* Princeton University Press, Princeton, New Jersey (1994)

Rosner, Fred, *Medicine In The Mishneh Torah Of Maimonides,* KTAV Publishing House, Inc., New York City, New York (1984)

Veatch, Robert M., *A Theory Of Medical Ethics,* Basic Books, Inc. Publishers, New York City, New York (1981)

When Death Is Sought. New York State Task Force On Life And The Law, New York City, New York (1994)

Wielenberg, Erik J., *Value And Virtue In A Godless Universe* (Cambridge University Press, New York City, New York (2005)

Wilson, James Q., *The Moral Sense* The Free Press, New York City, New York (1993)

NOTES

1. For a thorough exploration of this issue, see the excellent work by Sissela Bok called *Lying: Moral Choice in Public and Private Life*, Pantheon Books, New York City, New York, (1978).

2. Rodale, J.I. Revised by Urdang, Lawrence Editor in Chief, *The Synonym Finder*, Warner Books, Inc., New York City, New York, (1978).

3. AISSG (Androgen Insensitivity Syndrome Support Group), *www.medhelp.org/www/ais/*.

4. School Board of Nassau County, Florida, and Craig Marsh v. Gene H. Arline (1986), Thomas v. Atascadero Unified School District (1986), Ray v. School District of DeSoto County (1987), Doe v. Belleville Public School District No. 118 (1987).

5. Tarasoff v. Regents of the Univ. of Cal., 118 Cal. Rptr. 129 (Cal. 1974) (Tarasoff l) modified by Tarasoff v. Regents of the Univ. of Cal., 551 P. 2d 334 (Cal. 1976) (Tarasoff ll).

6. Pueschel, Siegfried M., M.D., *A Parent's Guide to Down Syndrome*, Paul H. Brooks Publishing Co., Inc., Baltimore, Maryland (2001).

7. National Down Syndrome Congress
    1370 Center Drive, Suite 102
    Atlanta, Georgia 30338
    Toll-free: 1-800-232-6372
    Email: info@ndsccenter.org
    Website: *www.ndsccenter.org*

    National Down Syndrome Society
    666 Broadway
    New York, New York 10012-2317
    Toll-free: 1-800-221-4602
    Email: info@ndss.org
    Website: *www.ndss.org*

National Dissemination Center for Children
with Disabilities (NICHY)
P.O. Box 1492
Washington, DC 20013
1-800-695-0285 · v/tty
1-202-884-8441 · fax
Email: nichcy@aed.org
Website: *www.nichcy.org*

8.   Reilly, Philip R., *The Surgical Solution: A History of Involuntary Sterilization in the United States,* Johns Hopkins Press, Baltimore, Maryland (1981).

9.   Colorado was not one of them, but only because of a gubernatorial veto.

10.   Philip R. Reilly, *The Surgical Solution: A History of Involuntary Sterilization in the United States* Johns Hopkins Press, Baltimore, Maryland (1981).

11.   Ibid.

12.   Buck v. Bell, 274 U.S. 200 (1927).

13.   Koontz, Claudia, *The Nazi Conscience,* Belknap Press of Harvard University, Cambridge, Massachusetts (2003).

Lifton, Robert J.,, *The Nazi Doctors,* Basic Books, Harper Collins, New York City, New York (1986).

14.   Skinner v. Oklahoma (1942) C729.

15.   Relf v. Weinberg, 372 F. Supp. 1196 (D.D.C. 1974) overturning federal regulations under which minor and incompetent poor persons had been involuntarily sterilized under federally financed family planning programs.

16.   In the Matter of A.W. 637 P.2d 366 (Colo. 1981).

17.   Sterilization of The Developmentally Disabled, Colorado Revised Statutes 27-10.5-128. 129. 130.

Sterilization is permitted for patients over
eighteen who consent, provided:

a.   She/he is competent to consent, consents freely and voluntarily as evaluated in the following way:

  1.   A psychiatrist, psychologist, or physician who does not provide services, and a developmental disabilities professional who does not provide services both consult with the surgeon concerning

their opinion regarding the validity of consent.

b. Both consult with the surgeon concerning their opinion regarding the validity of consent.

c. If the capacity of the person is challenged, she/he may petition a court to declare competency to consent.

　　1. The court will then appoint two or more experts in developmental disability to present their findings at a competency hearing.

　　2. If the court determines the person is competent and consents, the procedure may be done. If the patient is determined not to be competent, the procedure may not be done.

d. No one over eighteen who has the capacity to consent may be sterilized without consent.

Sterilization for Minors or Persons not Competent to Consent

a. A petition to the court includes:

　　1. the person's mental condition,

　　2. A statement of medical necessity to preserve life or health (mental or physical),

　　3. A statement why less intrusive methods would not serve the person's interests.

b. The court appoints an attorney to represent the person's interests and one or more experts in developmental disability to evaluate and testify regarding physical and mental findings and any relevant matters.

c. To order sterilization, the court must find:

　　1. The person lacks capacity or is a minor,

　　2. The court has heard and considered the person's desires,

　　3. The person lacks capacity and is unlikely to improve,

　　4. The person is capable of reproduction and is likely to be sexually active,

　　5. Clear and convincing evidence of medical necessity to preserve life or health (mental or physical).

　　6. Clear and convincing evidence why less intrusive methods would not serve the person's interests.

18. The ethics committee of The American College of Obstetricians and Gynecologists (ACOG) produced a committee opinion regarding "steril-

ization of women who are mentally handicapped" in 1988. It stated that decisions must be made in the best interests of the person for whom sterilization is proposed. It pointed out the many elements to consider in making the decision, among which were the types of consultants who would be sought for aid in evaluating consent and the appropriateness of the procedure. They also pointed out that "the presence of a mental handicap alone does not, in itself, justify either sterilization or its denial."

19. In 1999, the American Academy of Pediatrics updated their previous statement, also entitled "Sterilization of Women Who Are Mentally Handicapped," which had been published in 1990 as a companion to the above policy from the American College of Obstetricians and Gynecologists (*Pediatrics,* Vol. 104, No. 2, August 1999, pp. 337–340, "Sterilization of Minors with Developmental Disabilities"). It is a thoroughly referenced policy, again noting an increasing trend toward permitting as complete a life experience as possible for the developmentally disabled. To quote, "More recently, ethical precepts and public policy have emphasized the importance of providing the least restrictive life alternatives for persons with cognitive and other disabilities or disorders." Note that the mental disabilities were the same but their accepted names varied over the intervening years. The history of the eugenics movement and the backlash prohibiting sterilization are reviewed in the policy, and the caveats amplify and echo those of ACOG. Both warn practitioners to be cognizant of the widely varying state and federal regulations and laws.

20. Today, there is a quadruple screen that increases the ability to predict problems.

21. The joined egg and sperm is called an embryo by doctors up to eight weeks. After that, doctors call it a fetus until birth.

22. This citation and other quotations and cases to follow are found with references in the reports of The President's Commission for the Study of Ethical Problems in Medicine and Biomedical and Behavioral Research, *Making Healthcare Decisions,* Volume 3, *The Patient's Role in Medical Decision Making,* by Martin S. Pernick, Ph.D.

23. Schloendorff v. Society of New York Hospitals, 211 NY 125 N.E. 92 (1914).

24. Salgo v. Leland Stanford Jr. University 317 P 2nd 170 CAL 1st Dist. Ct. App. (1957).

25. Natanson v. Kline 186 Kan 392, 350 p,2d 1093 (1960).

26. Canterbury v. Spence 464 F 2d 772 (DC Cir (1972).

27. Lane v. Candura, 376 NE 2d 1232 (Mass. App. Ct. 1978).

28. Evidently, I was wrong and I have.

29. Meconium is fetal bowel content that appears as the anal sphincter relaxes with fetal distress.

30. A very carefully and completely referenced work of medical and political mistreatment of blacks in the United States throughout their long history is *Slavery, Segregation and Racism: Trusting the Health Care System Ain't Always Easy! An African American Perspective on Bioethics*, Vernellia R. Randall, 15 St. Louis University Public Law Review 191 1996 cite as 15 St. Louis U. Pub. L. Rev. 191 -235 (1996) The most notorious American experiment had begun before WW II. It concerned the failure to treat over four hundred black men for syphilis and simply, "observe the natural course of the disease"—as if centuries of observing the outcomes of syphilis had not clearly demonstrated this. The Tuskegee study began in 1933. Despite the availability of penicillin, the subjects continued to be followed without therapy until 1972. No one protested the study despite several papers that described it in scientific journals. Saddest of all, it was done under the auspices of the U.S. Public Health Service. Not until the second Clinton administration were an apology and reparations offered, too late for many who died or suffered the physical and mental ravages of the disease.

31. In January of 1983, 23 year old Nancy Cruzan was in a single car auto accident. She went without air for an estimated 12-14 minutes. Permanent brain damage occurs in 4-8 minutes. She was resuscitated at the scene, and never needed a ventilator to breath. Because she could not take food by mouth, a feeding tube was placed into her stomach through the abdominal wall in February. She never regained consciousness. She had a brain injury called the Permanent Persistent Vegetative State. After several years, her parents requested that the feeding tube be removed and Nancy be allowed to die. The Missouri trial court agreed. A court-appointed guardian ad litem for Nancy also agreed, but he joined the appeal so that a precedent in law could be established for future cases. It would become precedent only when it was affirmed at an appellate court level.

Everyone involved was surprised and disturbed when the Missouri Supreme Court reversed the decision, based upon the State interest in preserving life. They determined that only "clear and convincing evidence" of the patient's wishes could overcome the presumption.

In September 1990, the US Supreme Court gave their decision. Five justices recognized the right of a competent patient to refuse life-sustaining therapy. All agreed that the State had the right to set the level of evidence required for a *proxy* decision maker, to assure that the patient was truly represented. The principle is to err on the side of preserving life. The Court's decision was based neither on a finding of futility of treatment nor of greatly diminished quality of life, but upon the liberty-right of patients to self-determination—patient autonomy.

There was a retrial at the state level and the judge heard new evidence that Nancy, when an employee of a nursing home, had clearly stated to fellow employees that she would never wish to be sustained in the PVS like the patients for whom she was caring. The same court that first agreed the tube could be discontinued found this to be clear and convincing. The patient died about two weeks after tube feeding was discontinued. Reference to U.S. Supreme Court decision—Cruzan v. Director, Missouri Health Department 497 U.S. 261; 110 S.Ct. 2841; 111 L. Ed.2d 224 (1990).

32. Reich, Warren Thomas, Editor in Chief *Encyclopedia of Bioethics, revised edition*, V3, pp. 1420–1423, , Simon & Schuster Macmillan, New York City, New York (1995).

33. Cruzan v. Director, Missouri Health Department 497 U.S. 261; 110 S.Ct. 2841; 111 L. Ed.2d 224 (1990).

34. Vacco v. Quill, 117 S.Ct. 2293 (1997).

35. Satz v. Perlmutter, 362 So. 2d 160, 162-163 (Fla. App. 1978) .

36. Cruzan v. Director, Missouri Health Department 497 U.S. 261; 110 S.Ct. 2841; 111 L. Ed.2d 224 (1990).

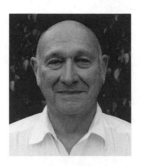

ABOUT THE AUTHOR

Fredrick R. Abrams, M.D., received his medical degree from Cornell University and for over forty years specialized in obstetrics and gynecology. At Rose Medical Center in Denver, he founded the first center for the study of ethical issues in a community-hospital setting in the U.S. As former chair of the Ethics Committee of the American College of Obstetricians and Gynecologists, he helped write the guidelines for its 25,000 members.

In 2003, the Department of Bioethics and Humanities of the University of Colorado Health Sciences Center presented him with a Lifetime Achievement Award, for "helping to create such a fertile ground for bioethics in Colorado." He is also the recipient of the 2006 Isaac Hays, M.D. and John Bell, M.D. Award for Leadership in Medical Ethics and Professionalism, presented by the American Medical Association.

Dr. Abrams has been published in *The New England Journal of Medicine*, *The Journal of the American Medical Association*, and many other periodicals.

He lives in Denver, Colorado.

Dr. Abrams is donating all the author profits from this book to the Center for Bioethics and Humanities at the University of Colorado Health Sciences Center.

Sentient Publications, LLC publishes books on cultural creativity, experimental education, transformative spirituality, holistic health, new science, and ecology, approached from an integral viewpoint. Our authors are intensely interested in exploring the nature of life from fresh perspectives, addressing life's great questions, and fostering the full expression of the human potential. Sentient Publications' books arise from the spirit of inquiry and the richness of the inherent dialogue between writer and reader.

We are very interested in hearing from our readers. To direct suggestions or comments to us, or to be added to our mailing list, please contact:

SENTIENT PUBLICATIONS, LLC
1113 Spruce Street
Boulder, CO 80302
303.443.2188
contact@sentientpublications.com
www.sentientpublications.com